What people are saying about

Going Nowhere, Slow

In this sharp and poetic book, Mikkel Krause Frantzen brilliantly illustrates the horror of depression. But he doesn't leave us there, in despair, but opens up new hopeful ways of thinking about the spirit of our time.

Carl Cederström, author of *The Happiness Fantasy*, and co-author of *Dead Man Working, The Wellness Syndrome*, and *Desperately Seeking Self-Improvement*

Why are we all so depressed? Today, depression is less an individual malady, than it is a structure of feeling that pervades Western neoliberal society. In this book, Mikkel Krause Frantzen digs deeply into this situation, reading a number of works (novels, movies, visual art) that not only give expression to our depressive condition, but offer clues as to why and how we feel this way.

Steven Shaviro, author of *The Cinematic Body, Connected, or What It Means to Live in the Network Society, The Universe of Things*, and *Discognition*

In this groundbreaking book, Mikkel Krause Frantzen takes depression as something that does not simply have connection with the subject's past and alienation from others, but also to the idea of future and too much closeness. As a result, Frantzen finds in depression glimmers of optimism and hope. This book is essential reading for anyone who has questioned what depression is all about and why so many well-known novelists have created their best works trying to come to grips with it.

Renata Salecl, author of *Tyranny of Choice, (Per)versions of love and hate*, and *On anxiety*

Going Nowhere, Slow

The Aesthetics and Politics
of Depression

Going Nowhere, Slow

The Aesthetics and Politics
of Depression

Mikkel Krause Frantzen

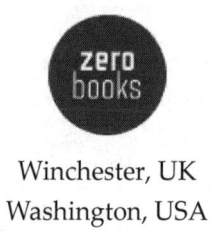

Winchester, UK
Washington, USA

JOHN HUNT PUBLISHING

First published by Zero Books, 2019
Zero Books is an imprint of John Hunt Publishing Ltd., No. 3 East St., Alresford,
Hampshire SO24 9EE, UK
office@jhpbooks.com
www.johnhuntpublishing.com
www.zero-books.net

For distributor details and how to order please visit the 'Ordering' section on our website.

Text copyright: Mikkel Krause Frantzen 2018

ISBN: 978 1 78904 214 6
978 1 78904 215 3 (ebook)
Library of Congress Control Number: 2018961090

A CIP catalogue record for this book is available from the British Library.

Design: Stuart Davies

UK: Printed and bound by CPI Group (UK) Ltd, Croydon, CR0 4YY
US: Printed and bound by Thomson-Shore, 7300 West Joy Road, Dexter, MI 48130

We operate a distinctive and ethical publishing philosophy in
all areas of our business, from our global network of authors to
production and worldwide distribution.

Contents

Prologue (two questions)

Two absolutely quotidian questions somehow form the basis of the present work, which studies the psychopathology of depression in the Western world today, through the examination of four cultural works: the fiction of Michel Houellebecq, the fiction of David Foster Wallace, the installation and video works of the artistic duo who sign their collaborations under the name of Claire Fontaine, and finally Lars von Trier's film *Melancholia*.

The first very simple question is the one that we, innocently, ask and answer every day: How are you? How is it going? Nowhere do we get a better description of the banality and brutality of this question than in the book *Suicide* (2008) by French author and artist Édouard Levé. In this book, which he handed over to his editor a couple of weeks before he took his own life in 2007, Levé conjures up the suicide of a depressed childhood friend 20 years earlier. The book is a work of fiction, written in the second person, as a continuous address to this childhood friend and an incessant reflection upon his life and death, though it is impossible not to read the book as some sort of self-portrait (which, incidentally, was the title of one of Levé's previous books). In this book, the following scene appears:

One evening you were invited to dine at a friend's house with other guests. To the host who, opening the door for you on your arrival, asked you how you were doing, you responded, "Badly." [...] You didn't want to disrupt the party, but you couldn't make yourself lie in response to the simple question, "How are you doing?" You were more honest than courteous. Even though you were capable of it, it seemed unthinkable to you to put on a show of well-being for a close friend. Having arrived in the living room, you did not want to reproduce the unease sparked by your first response. To your friend's

1

friends, some of whom you didn't know, you presented a friendly exterior. In this atmosphere, which made you feel foreign, you were surprised at your own success in putting on the appropriate face, which, if it didn't contribute to the general euphoria, at least didn't destroy the mood with its indifference.[1]

This question – how are you doing? – is as banal as it is brutal, as predictable as it is profound. And in a situation like the one outlined in Levé's book, it appears that it is imperative to lie, since to answer this question in earnest would involve breaking every possible code of conduct: Well, you see, not so well, I feel depressed, I cannot get up in the morning, my wife has just left me, my boss is an idiot, my life is meaningless etc. But most people do not do that, they prefer to keep the spirits high and the atmosphere nice and cozy. So, they lie, or, they just refrain from telling the truth, they say: I am fine, thank you very much. And how are you by the way?

The second question, equally banal, is: What time is it? What is the time? At a bar called Lygtens Kro in Copenhagen, a sign is hanging on the wall amidst old-fashioned ornaments and stall cigarette smoke. It says: "The one who is happy does not notice that time goes by" (in Danish: Den som er lykkelig lægger ikke mærke til at tiden går). An unhappy person, a depressed person, on the other hand, is all too painfully aware of the passing of time. In this state seconds crawl forward, they drag themselves along. Following the course taken by the matter itself, I make the case in this book that the abortion of the future that occurs in depression entails that all that remains is a kind of eternal present full of pain and horror, and the feeling that this is all there is, always has been and always will be.

"It's like horror more than sadness. It's more like horror," says the clinically depressed Kate Gompert in David Foster Wallace's *Infinite Jest* from 1996. "I can't stand feeling like this

2

another second, and the seconds keep coming on and on." And in Michel Houellebecq's novels, especially in his debut novel *Whatever* from 1994, the depressed protagonists thus always know what time it is. It is 2 in the afternoon. It is 6.20. Here, time has become thoroughly explicit in the same way as Heidegger says that we only notice any given tool – a hammer, for instance – at that moment when it does not work anymore. In depression, time becomes elastic, it becomes explicit, then it snaps.

In this book *Going Nowhere, Slow – the Aesthetics and Politics of Depression*, these two questions are inextricably linked. What time is it and how are you? These are the questions that every depressed person dislikes and fears. In fact, to the depressed person there is no difference between them; they remain one and the same. Also, these questions are not purely personal, psychological questions. They are also and perhaps above all deeply political questions. This book, intended as a diagnosis of the times, hinges upon these questions of time and effect. In other words: In order to answer the question *what kind of times are these?* we can simply, I contend, ask the depressed person *what time is it?* Only then do we really get a sense of the present state of affairs. But as a literary scholar and cultural theorist my method is not quantitative: I have not formulated any questionnaires to be answered by one of the now 300 million people who are estimated to suffer from depression according to a new report from the World Health Organization (WHO). What I have done instead is ask some exemplary depressed art works the same questions. What time is it? How is it going?

Introduction

Welcome to the world's happiest nation

If you traveled to Denmark in the fall of 2015 you were likely greeted by Carlsberg, welcoming you not only to Copenhagen Airport, but to the world's happiest nation. Or so the advert read: Welcome to the world's happiest nation. From the way the message was presented, it was clear that the statement was not supposed to be doubted, or read ironically. From a certain point of view, it is simply the plain truth, an objective fact that can be measured and proved: *The World Happiness Report* consistently ranks the Danes as one of the happiest peoples in the world. Yet, as the Danish Mental Health Foundation makes clear, more and more Danes are diagnosed with depression: At any given time, 4 to 5 percent of the population is depressed, or, more accurately, diagnosed as such. Indeed, according to the Danish Health Authority more than 450,000 Danes bought anti-depressants in 2011, a figure which has almost doubled over the past decade.

This tendency can be observed all over the Western world. The US National Institute of Mental Health estimates that 9.5 percent of the adult American population – 18.8 million people – suffers from depression. These numbers have led the WHO to conclude that depression is the most common mental disorder and the prime cause of disability and suicide, affecting around 350 million people worldwide. No wonder, then, that the consumption of SSRI-antidepressants has gone through the roof with sales now approaching 6 billion dollars annually.

These facts and figures seem to speak for themselves, but it is necessary to remember that the sale of anti-depressants does not correspond exactly to occurrences of depression, as SSRIs are not exclusively used for treating depression, but purchased to treat a range of other mental illnesses as well. Moreover, the frequency of diagnoses does not necessarily mirror the frequency of depressions, so that one might wonder if the increase in diagnoses testifies to a growing number of depressed people or rather to an escalating tendency to pathologize common, "normal" affects such as sadness and grief, translating them into the diagnostic category of depression.

Regardless, it seems quite clear that depression has developed into a paradigm and remains the prevalent psychopathology of our time with all the moral, economic and political implications that this entails. Allan V. Horwitz and Jerome C. Wakefield write, in *The Loss of Sadness*, that "depression has gained an iconic status in both the contemporary mental health professions and the culture at large."[1] We see it in TV-shows such as *The Sopranos* (1999-2007) and *Happyish* (2015), dramatic plays such as *All my dreams come true* by Christian Lollike (2013/14), the interactive computer game *Depression Quest* (2013), contemporary art exhibitions such as *Depression* (2009, Marres, Maastricht) and *Unendlicher Spass* (2014, Schirn, Frankfurt), documentary films like *The Dark Gene* (2015) and book publications ranging from nonfiction work *The Noonday Demon: An Atlas of Depression* by Andrew Solomon (2001), to poetry collections such as *i am a little bit happier than you are* by American poet Tao Lin (2006) or the aformentioned *Suicide* by Édouard Levé (2008).

For this reason alone, it seems relevant to examine the relation between depression and contemporary literature, arts, movies and "culture at large." It seems necessary for a cultural analysis that claims a certain criticality and contemporaneity to dwell on scenes of unhappiness and, more specifically, depression. This is what I do in this book, through analysis of books by David Foster Wallace and Michel Houellebecq, works by the ready-made artist Claire Fontaine and the movie *Melancholia* by Lars von Trier. In this way, *Going Nowhere, Slow* is conceived as a way of contributing to the cultural analysis of the present, a *Zeitdiagnose* as the Germans would say, with the important caveat that it is the works' own diagnoses of the times that are the focus of attention.

The underlying premise is that there is no better way to understand the psychopathology of depression than to relate it to the problem of time, i.e. to understand depression in temporal terms, more specifically as a problem of futurity. I thus view depression as the pathological feeling that history has come to an end, that the future is closed off, frozen once and for all. Based on a method that I call scenographic symptomatology, which means simply that the book is built around specific scenes with an accompanying set of symptoms, all of the chapters are variations on this personal, political if not planetary problem of futurity.

What do we talk about when we talk about depression?

What do we talk about when we talk about depression? How do we define it and capture its specificity? How do we deal with this phenomenon without treating it merely as a conglomerate of other previously known mental illnesses such as anxiety, panic, melancholia, tiredness, boredom, sadness and so on? Water consists of hydrogen and oxygen but is in no way exhausted by this definition, which gives us little idea of the nature of water. In the same way depression seems to consist of and include components from some or all of the above-mentioned phenomena. And yet there is something more to depression, something specific that makes it discrete and distinguishable from other related phenomena. This is why the definition of depression advanced by the influential Diagnostic and Statistical Manual of Mental Disorders (DSM), which lists a set of symptoms such as tiredness, insomnia, suicidal impulses etc., is not comprehensive let alone satisfactory, though perhaps understandable from a practical, clinical point of view.

The concept of depression has always been haunted by

classificatory problems: From Freud, who in his famous text "Mourning and Melancholia" (1917) observed that the empirical foundation for defining melancholia leaves something to be desired, to Ludwig Binswanger, who in the book *Melancholie und Manie* (1960) expressed similar concerns, prompting him to avoid the concept altogether, since, as he wrote, it had so many disparate and heterogeneous meanings and appeared to be so washed-out that it could no longer form the basis of a real scientific investigation. Today this conceptual haziness has still not abated. Depression is, as Christine Ross writes, "the slippery notion par excellence of psychiatry."[2] It would be an exaggeration to speak of a diagnostic chaos, but the only thing people seem to agree is that they cannot agree on a definition of depression. Is depression a chemical imbalance in the brain? Is it biologically or socially determined? Is it caused by genes or the environment, is it a nervous problem affecting the whole body rather than a problem of mood and affect? Is it to be distinguished sharply from normal sadness? Is it somewhat similar to the black bile of melancholy – the ancient concept of *melaina chole* as one of the four humors – or more akin to the medieval notion of spiritual *acedia*? Is it an illness, something abnormal and pathological, or is it a "normal" and "healthy" reaction to an abnormal and unhealthy society? What is it?

Going Nowhere, Slow rests on the supposition that depression is a chronopathology, characterized by the loss of (the ability to imagine) the future. Not the loss of a precise future but precisely the loss of future itself. This is a controversial or at least unconventional standpoint, viewed in the context of diagnostic manuals like the DSM, in which time or temporal experience does not feature among the otherwise extensive list of depressive symptoms. However, within phenomenological psychiatry and philosophy things there are plenty of discussions of the relation of depression and time. In his *General Psychopathology*, Karl Jaspers, who was not just a philosopher but also a psychiatrist, is interested in the experience of time in mental disorders. According to the anthropology of the phenomenological tradition that has Husserl and Heidegger as its founding fathers, to be a human being is to be a temporal being with a direction, a sense of continuity, and some plan for the future (what Husserl called *protention* and Heidegger conceptualized as the ec-static temporality of being, the anticipation of future possibilities). But this, as Jaspers points out, is precisely what depressed patients lack: After quoting a depressive patient complaining that, "it feels as if it is always the same moment, it is like a timeless void," Jaspers comments: "A depressed patient feels as if time did not want to go on."[3] To Jaspers, this experience or awareness of time is intimately connected to an emotional atmosphere in that emotional changes make themselves noticeable in the experience of time:

> A depressed patient, suffering from "terrible emptiness" and a feeling of "having lost all feeling" reported – "I cannot see the future, just as if there were none. I think everything is going to stop now and tomorrow there will be nothing at all." Patients know there is another day tomorrow but this awareness has changed from what it was like before. Even the next five minutes do not lie ahead as they used to do. Such patients have no decisions, no worries, no hopes for the future.[4]

Jaspers even develops the fruitful idea of what could be called a meta-feeling, in particular the idea of the feeling of a non-feeling (*Gefühl der Gefühllosigkeit* or *Fühlen eines Nichtfühlen*), so that in depression one feels nothing, but this feeling of nothing is definitely felt. Or to put it another way: the feeling of not feeling anything is itself a feeling. This is not sheer sophistry, but rather the ultimate – affective – horror of depression, which will become clear in the case of David Foster Wallace. In any case, it becomes crucial to explore not just depression as a feeling, but how that feeling feels; what depression feels like.[5]

In the words of German psychiatrist and philosopher Thomas Fuchs, a desynchronization occurs in depression that is as social as it is biological. Normally, Fuchs says, we do not pay any attention to time, we just live in it. But in depression this is no longer the case. In this type of situation, time is suddenly *noticed*: it becomes perceptively and painfully out of joint, out of synch.[6] In fact, several studies show that depression is the excruciating feeling of being stuck, stagnated; that it feels like the race is run, like the present – which is hell – is all there is and all that can ever be imagined to be. These studies are filled with people who describe depression as a vacuum, as a room with no windows and no doors, as an icecold ocean, or as flames that burn the subject alive.[7] Some compare depression with falling, with losing your footing, some note that being depressed is similar to being a zombie, a living dead. What unites these descriptions and metaphors is that there is no hope and imagination in depression. In the state of depression, you have no hope for the future, you cannot imagine the depression – except, perhaps, in dystopic colors. In other words: The future is considered a thing of the past, a *fait accompli*. Somewhere in his book on depression, *Time and Inner Future,* the American psychiatrist Frederick T. Melges quotes a patient who describes how "the future looks cold and bleak, and I seem frozen in time"; it is as if a cloud has drawn "a curtain on the future."[8]

The point in *Going Nowhere, Slow* is that a curtain has also been drawn on the future in a more general, historical and political sense, not least as far as the societies of the Western world are concerned. Here, the phenomenological tradition reaches its limits for my present purposes. Though it offers a nuanced and empirical understanding of depression as a temporal psychopathology, it remains inadequate as a means to address depression as a *political* problem. The phenomenological literature must be supplemented by certain contemporary political theories, which, in turn, can and must be supported by the empirical basis that has just been described in order that this more speculative mode of thought does not melt into air.

There is no alternative (old wine in new bottles?)

There is a lot of merit to Franco "Bifo" Berardi's analysis of depression as a symptom of a society that has lost (the ability to imagine) the future. In later works such as *After the Future* (2011) and *The Uprising. On Poetry and Finance* (2012), he presents the argument that the current crisis is not so much an economic, social or political crisis as a crisis in the imagination of the future. The promise of the future – so present and clear at the beginning of the twentieth century in the work of the avant-garde, the Futurists and so on – has now evaporated: "The future no longer appears as a choice or a collective conscious action, but is a kind of unavoidable catastrophe that we cannot oppose in any way."[9] For Berardi the decisive year was 1977, a foreboding of what was and perhaps still is to come: "The end of modernity began with the collapse of the future, with Sid Vicious screaming *no future.*"[10] This historical situation must therefore, according to Berardi, be related to the emergence and proliferation of a psychopathology such as depression:

> The future becomes a threat when the collective imagination becomes incapable of seeing alternatives to trends leading to devastation, increased poverty, and violence. This is precisely our current situation, because capitalism has become a system of techno-economic automatisms that politics cannot evade. The paralysis of the will (the impossibility of politics) is the historical context of today's depression epidemic.[11]

In his book *Ghosts of My Life. Writings on Depression, Hauntology and Lost Futures* (2012), the late Mark Fisher picks up the thread from Berardi in his attempt to apprehend that the future is not what it used to be. When Fisher talks about hauntology, a concept he borrows from Jacques Derrida's writing on Marx's ghosts, he alludes to the idea that the present seems to be haunted by the future – *in its very absence*. This specter of an absent future constitutes a kind of hauntology in reverse: It is a hauntology *from* the future, not from the past; a hauntology *of* a lost future. *Ghosts of My Life* is thus not only the natural successor to the work of Berardi, but also to Fisher's own book *Capitalist Realism* (2009), in which Fisher – informed, also, by the work of Fredric Jameson – conceptualizes "the widespread sense that not only is capitalism the only viable political and economic system, but also that it is now impossible even to imagine a coherent alternative to it."[12] He calls this widespread sense *capitalist realism*. As an epitomization of "the spectres of lost futures,"[13] depression can be viewed as the pathological mirror of contemporary capitalism; there is a strange resonance between capitalist realism and "the deflationary perspective of a depressive who believes that any positive state, any hope, is a dangerous illusion."[14]

One question that does not concern Fisher is where this leaves the hypothesis of depressive realism, which states that depressed persons are not depressed because they have a distorted or delusional view of reality, but because they have a more accurate perception of reality than people who are not depressed. Within psychology the notion of depressive realism emerged from an infamous study conducted in 1979 by Alloy and Abramson, but Freud had already pointed out that depressed people have "a keener eye for the truth than others who are not melancholic" and that "we only wonder why a man has to be ill before he can be accessible to a truth of this kind."[15] In *Going Nowhere, Slow,* I seek to challenge and complicate this particular notion of depressive realism throughout. On the one hand, it is imperative to avoid the *pathologization* of depression found in diagnostic manuals and biomedical psychiatry. On the other, it is essential to sidestep the kind of *romanticizing* that is inherent to the idea of depressive realism.

To get back to the main thread of the argument and confront the series of questions regarding periodization that have emerged so far. Given the fact that depression has been on the rise for several decades now and, in a way, is our historical present, it becomes a question of periodizing this present. "We cannot not periodize," as Fredric Jameson famously wrote in *A Singular Modernity*.[16] In general, I think we must be wary of broad and generalized claims about the transitions from modernity to postmodernity, from one temporal regime to the next. That said, it seems beyond doubt that the idea of progress so prominent during the better part of the twentieth century has more or less faded today, and that a historical transition has taken place that is inextricably bound up with the emergence of depression as the topical psychopathology of our time: A transition from modernity to postmodernity, from Fordism to Post-fordism, from a society of prohibition and discipline to a post-disciplinary society of autonomy and control.

The phenomenon of depression can – and indeed ought to – be related to a (Western) world which has arrived at the end of history, in the sense that there is no alternative, as Margaret Thatcher triumphantly declared decades ago. The crisis embodied by depression thus becomes a symptom of a more general crisis of futurity. Following Berardi and Fisher, it seems impossible to separate the history of depression from the societal and historical changes that emerged in the wake of 1968 and accelerated during the economic crisis of the 1970s, leading in the end to a neoliberal[17] restructuring of the global economy. Historical development since then, with low growth rates, declining or stagnant real wages, structural unemployment, privatization or outsourcing of public services, the steady precarization of labor markets all around the world, a brutal debilitation of unions, explosive financialization and deregulation of the economy, culminated in 2008 with thorough-going crisis. However, the crisis is by no means over and done with, not least due to the fact that austerity measures and a politics of necessity have been considered the sole solutions to the crisis and the only available means of moving forward, which is to say: Going nowhere at all (though it has created an enormous increase in private as well as public debt). There is no point to question whether or not this is a neoliberal development in its most exemplary form. German sociologist Wolfgang Streeck is adamant that it is: "The present financial, fiscal and economic crisis is the end point so far of the long neoliberal transformation of postwar capitalism."[18] In this context I can only hint at some concrete events and decisive dates in this transformation, that include but are not limited to: The abolition of the Bretton Woods system of international financial exchange and the cancellation of the convertibility of the US dollar to gold in 1971; the oil crisis of 1973; Thatcher's election as prime minister of the UK in 1979; the appointment of Paul Volcker as chairman of the US Federal Reserve Bank in October of the same year; and the inauguration of Ronald Reagan as US president in 1980. The rest is (neoliberal) history.

The fall of the Berlin Wall in 1989 only made manifest what was, in a sense, already an established reality: The end of history. A post-historical, post-modern and post-political situation, in which *time is no more* (as it is proclaimed in the apocalypse). No coincidence, then, that one of the last sentences of Michel Houellebecq's novel *The Possibility of an Island* reads: "The future was empty."[19] In fact, all the works discussed in this book are primarily oriented toward the future, or, more precisely, toward a future that is not there, a future that is already lost.

But is this loss of the future, a loss which is simultaneously a personal and a political problem, not simply the – by now almost ancient – problem of postmodernism? Is it not just old wine in new bottles? Yes and no. The new or contemporary feature of the no-future *stimmung* that writers such as Jameson (and Lyotard) addressed quite a long time ago – emphatically encapsulated by Jameson's famous quip that it is easier to imagine the end of the world than an alternative to capitalism – is that, today, this is no longer the shocking realization of a cultural vanguard such as the punk movement. At most it generates a shrug of the shoulders and a concomitant: So what? What *was* originally a diffuse albeit perceptive intuition, has now become a habit; what only existed in an embryonic form, something in the air, has now become a generalized, naturalized and almost common condition. In that respect, the future is not what it used to be. This seems to be the backdrop to the phenomenon of depression today.

What also separates our age from earlier times is that alienation has assumed a different character. The problem nowadays is not a homogenous, mechanical and monotonous time, but a heterogeneous, flexible and momentary time; people are not reduced to objects – dehumanized creatures on assembly lines – but rather produced as subjects. Unlike the alienation of yesterday, which always implied *distance,* an abyss between man and machine, between animate subjectivity and sterile temporality, alienation today seems characterized by *proximity* and *immersion.* The problem, it appears, is that one has become so integral a part of the (net)work that – the moment it is no longer possible to keep up – one implodes rather than explodes; not hitting one's head against a brick wall, but collapsing down into the hole at the very heart of the contemporary capitalist machinery. "We are depressed not because we are so far removed from what we want, but because we are merged with it."[20] In many ways, *Going Nowhere, Slow* is a story about this contemporary form of alienation.[21]

For these particular reasons do I speak of depression and not melancholia. Of course, the mental illness has been known since the dawn of time, and there is a rich tradition of both medical texts and works of art stretching all the way back to Hippocrates and Aristotle. Some core aspects of the disease may not have changed, some of the symptoms may indeed be immutable and eternal. But the historical context in which it unfolds is not. Its status and significance vary, so do the causes and effects. In his book *The Weariness of the Self. Diagnosing the History of Depression in the Contemporary Age* (2010), perhaps the most influential sociological study of depression so far, Alain Ehrenberg argues that depression separates itself from melancholia after the Second World War, not least due to the fact that it was at that time that the transition from a disciplinary society to a more post-disciplinary regime took place. In this latter regime people are not judged in terms of obedience but in terms of autonomy, that is to say, in terms of each individual's ability to perform, to network, to be entrepreneurial, to demonstate initiative and to realize themselves.[22] It is a society within which the fantasy of the good, authentic and happy life developed into a normative demand, at once institutionalized at a societal level and internalized at a personal level. It is a society in which the central question is not "am I allowed to do it?", but "am I able to do it?" According to Ehrenberg, melancholia has traditionally been associated with aristocracy and the idea of the exceptional man, disposed to both madness and creativity, which is not only observed by Michelangelo, but also and above all by Aristotle some 2 millennia earlier. Depression, on the other hand, is for everybody and not the "prerogative" of men, aristocrats and artists. As Susan Sontag remarked in *Illness as Metaphor*: Depression is melancholy – minus its charm. It is this charmless illness that this book is an attempt to understand.

Scenographic symptomatology (or you're probably so depressed and exhausted by now that you can't be bothered to read this)

How can one write about depression without falling into depressed speech, and without standing outside and remaining unaffected by what one is writing about? As Bernard Stiegler writes: "Speaking about misery always entails exposing oneself to the risk of becoming miserable [...] it is only possible to speak of *that which affects the miserable* to the extent that one finds *oneself affected* in one way or the other."[23] Placing oneself outside of the subject is not a viable solution, as Stiegler also points out. Becoming affected by and entangled in the empirical material is not merely an option but a condition. There is no way out, no other way about it. Yet, the task is – at the same time – one of finding a position in relation to depression or developing a discourse on depression that is not in itself depressing.[24]

By the same token, Lauren Berlant has pointed out that at one point she began to write from:

> the position of depressive realism in which the world's hard scenes ride the wave of the optimism inscribed in ambivalence, but without taking on optimism's conventional tones. I do not have the aim of moving beyond x but the aim of sitting there awhile, dedramatizing the performance of critical and political judgment so as to slow down the encounter with the objects of knowledge that are really scenes we can barely get our eyes around.[25]

Notwithstanding the fact that I, as stated previously, do not subscribe to the theory of depressive realism, I readily accept the challenge that Berlant puts on the table. Slowing down "the encounter with the objects of knowledge," is thus elevated to a methodological principle precisely because it allows for surprise encounters and for following the unexpected twists and turns in any given scene. I would indeed say, then, that this study of the relation between depression and contemporary culture within a temporal framework is a study that is based on what I call a scenographic symptomatology not only in terms of the mode of presentation but also in terms of its mode of inquiry. In plain words this means that each chapter of this book is built around specific scenes of literature, art and film. But there is a little more to it than that.

The scene forces an analytical approach which in this context can be translated into a principle of pausing and lingering at the individual scenes of depression, which are admittedly circular, but also open, not least to each other: They circle around themselves, around each other and around their already ever-empty centers. There is not, then, one coherent, linear argument, but rather a series of scenes, a series of arguments. The dramaturgy of the book thus seeks to avoid a narrative of progress(ion) in favor of a more paratactic technique, which involves hesitant, lateral and crab-like movements. As a consequence, one is forced to look at – or rather listen to – the *Klagen* and *Anklagen* that arise as an echo out of the abyss of depression in the individual scenes.

It was Freud who, in "Mourning and Melancholia," engaged in a speculation on the complaints (*Klagen*) and accusations (*Anklagen*) of the melancholic patient. But *Going Nowhere, Slow* turns Freud's argument upside down. To Freud the *Klagen* and *Anklagen* were always directed inwards, toward the melancholic self, as part of the endless production of narcissistic guilt and excessive self-hatred of melancholy, meaning that everything evolved around what the melancholic subject *in reality* said about his or her self. Here, in contrast, it is more a question of mapping out and trying to understand what this same self has to say *about reality*. How the world appears from the position and perspective of depression and what the depressive subject is really talking about when she is talking about herself – those are the questions. In relation to literary texts, for example, one important implication is that the attention must not only be directed toward any given text's view of depression, but also toward the view of the world that the depressive experience occasions in the work in question.

Accordingly, the analytical task requires at least two more or less explicit steps: As a first step, it is a matter of localizing and specifying the depressive experience (a constellation of symptoms), and, as a second step, of perceiving this experience as a response to a problem, or, as may well be the case, the actual production of a given problem (an articulation of conflict, a process of problematization). The questions then become: What kinds of – contemporary and social – problems do the works of art, not merely respond to but also, to a certain extent, produce? How do they respond? Can the response be said to be some sort of "therapeutic" cure, to perform a certain pharmacological function? How critical and how clinical can depressive art claim to be, in other words? How do they avoid being purely pessimistic pieces of art, seduced by the cynicism that seems to be an almost inevitable affective attendant to the pathology of depression?

Such questions animate the four chapters on the French writer Michel Houellebecq, the American author David Foster Wallace, the artist duo Claire Fontaine, and Danish film director Lars von Trier's *Melancholia*. Four chapters, four variations on the problem of futurity, four sets of symptoms or constellation of symptoms, and four specific problems, or articulations of cultural and political conflicts: Competition in Houellebecq, addiction in Wallace, debt in Claire Fontaine, happiness/the end of the world in von Trier. And also, four responses, four pharmacological models, which can tentatively and rather roughly be schematized as follows: If Houellebecq's response is techno-scientific and pertains to a transgression of being human, Wallace's is ethico-spiritual and pertains to a recovery of the other, Claire Fontaine's is radical-political and pertains to a transformation of depression into a strike, and von Trier's is cosmic-eschatological and pertains to the erection of an architecture of hope against all evidence to the contrary.

Chapter 1

The future was empty – Michel Houellebecq

Introduction

There is not a single protagonist in the novels of Houellebecq who is not depressed. From his debut novel *Extension du domaine de la lutte* (mysteriously translated as *Whatever*) to his latest *Soumission* (*Submission*), from the nameless narrator in the former to François in the latter, a depressive experience seems to saturate every fiber, every word. Descending into a specific scene from *Whatever*, I begin this chapter by analyzing the constellation of depressive symptoms, primarily expressed in the book as a problem of futurity.

If this first scene involves an investigation into the articulation of depression in *Whatever* as a problem – an investigation of the experience of depression in its own right – the subsequent scenes gradually shift focus toward how the experience of depression in turn articulates – or is symptomatic of – some pertinent problems in the historical context within which this experience arises and unfolds. Bearing in mind the previous modification of Freud's distinction between the melancholic *Klagen* and *Anklagen*, I stipulate that the *Anklagen* voiced in the works of Houellebecq are aimed at the twin trajectories of neoliberalism and May 1968, whose two ideologies of (economic) competition and (erotic) liberation have converged in the figure of the entrepreneur, and resulted in an expanded field of battle within which it has become impossible to distinguish between money and sex. In this chapter I am, in other words, tracing the movement from a phenomenological experience of depression to depression's problematization of the political economy. Or perhaps, rather than a movement from the former to the latter, I should describe it as an oscillation between the two, insofar as it is more an analytical distinction than an actual relation. In practice – i.e. in Houellebecq's *oeuvre* as whole – the two levels are inseparable. Perhaps one could even speak of his depressive literature as a phenomenology of the political economy?

Venturing into an analysis of *Les particules élémentaires* (*Atomised*), scene two looks at Houellebecq's critique of the political economy, his diagnosis of the times as formulated from and through the depressive experience laid bare in scene one. After that, in scenes three and four, I attend to two possible models of cure to be found in Houellebecq's body of work. Dealing with *La possibilité d'une* île (*The Possibility of an Island*) – a novel which in a sense is a sequel to *Atomised* – scene three is concerned with the question of science and technology, whereas scene four, which offers a reading of *Submission*, takes up the question of religion and spirituality. But what about art and literature in Houellebecq's pharmacological *experimentarium*? The quite extensive outro (or threshold as I have chosen to call it) will serve as an opportunity to ponder this question. It may well be that literature – like philosophy according to Simon Critchley – begins with a disappointment, but who is to say whether it might not also be interested in ending in one?

Scene 1. Pizza, porn and pills (*Whatever*)

> From time to time, he [the psychiatrist] glances at his wristwatch (fawn leather strap, rectangular gold-plated face); I get the feeling of not overly interesting him. I ask myself if he keeps a revolver in his drawer, for patients in a state of violent crisis. At the end of half an hour he pronounces a few phrases of general import on periods of blankness, extends my leave of absence and increases my dosage of medication. He also reveals that my condition has a name: it's a depression. Officially, then, I'm in a depression. The formula seems a happy one to me. It's not that I feel tremendously low; it's rather that the world around me appears high.[1]

Here he is, the protagonist and narrator of Michel Houellebecq's debut novel *Whatever* from 1994. The man without a name is a computer programmer, he is 30 years old but feels much older, and his life consists of nothing but pizza, porn and pills. He is clearly unhappy, but why does the formula – that he is in a depression – seem a happy one to him? What does it mean that rather than feeling low, he feels that the world around him is high? What kind of topography is that? And what sort of realism is at work here and in the novel as a whole?

"Failure, everywhere failure"

It is not until the very expiration of *Whatever* that the narrator receives the diagnosis of depression, but from beginning to end he exhibits a variety of depressive symptoms. He is inactive, immobilized, utterly exhausted and without any interest whatsoever in material things, social interaction, erotic adventures or life in general. He is incapable of investing his desire in "the possibility of establishing various interconnections between individuals, projects, organizations, service."[2] He is totally disinvested, completely disconnected.

At one point, he is on a business trip somewhere in France: He wants to go to Paris, he buys a ticket, he waits for the train, he does not go. This is, in so many words, a perfect example of the pathology of action integral to depression. The protagonist in *Whatever* can go back to Paris or he can stay where he is: It does not make any difference. But if one is unable to act oneself, one can certainly attempt to get others to act on one's behalf. In the depressive state of affairs that makes up his life, every action is outsourced. He is, however, not alone on this business trip but accompanied by a man called Raphael Tisserand, a sad little frog-like virgin in his late twenties. At Christmas time the two of them decide to celebrate by going to a disco. Raphael tries to pick up one woman after the other but to no avail. One woman in particular, or more precisely a young girl, catches his attention and when she leaves with – in the deliberately inappropriate jargon of the novel – a "mulatto," the narrator and Raphael follow them down to a beach. The secret plan of the former is to persuade the latter to kill the man and, afterwards, the girl (a scene obviously alluding to Albert Camus' *The stranger*). The point is that the depressed protagonist outsources the main and central act, except that it never takes place: Raphael does in fact go down to the beach, but instead of using his knife to kill the couple who are now having sex, he jerks off. He then drags himself back to the car, says goodbye to the narrator, gets in, drives off toward Paris and is killed in an accident on the way home. The chain of events has something overtly ridiculous and comical about it. To quote Beckett: "Nothing is funnier than unhappiness." It would, however, be a mistake to claim that the laughter in Houellebecq has a redemptive function. In the end, every comedian – and Houellebecq is a comedian, no doubt about it, even if, or rather because, his literature is so depressive – must come to realize that life, as a line goes in *The Possibility of an Island*, "fundamentally *is not* comical."[3]

Back in *Whatever*, New Year's Eve is coming up: "I walk from place to place in the grip of a fury, needing to act, yet can do nothing about it because any attempt seems doomed in advance. Failure, everywhere failure. Only suicide hovers above me, gleaming and inaccessible," the narrator states.[4] Suicide is not an option either: He is too depressed and impotent for that too. And then he is hospitalized.

What is up and what is down? The topography of depression

The scene at the psychiatric clinic where the narrator and protagonist receives his diagnosis is strangely reminiscent of Søren Kierkegaard's description of despair in *Sickness unto Death*, published under the pseudonym Anti-Climacus in 1849. In this book Kierkegaard develops a regular typology of despair, the conceptual pair most relevant for my purposes being his description of a despair of possibility and a despair of necessity. In a situation of excess of possibility the self, Kierkegaard writes, "flounders around in possibility until it is exhausted," whereas in a situation of too little possibility "a person seems unable to breathe."[5] Despite the very self-conscious mockery of Hegelian dialectics throughout – nowhere clearer than in the famous opening lines where the self is defined as spirit, that is as a relation that relates itself to itself – there *is* a dialectical tinge to the concept of despair. According to Kierkegaard, in some cases there can even be something diabolical or demonic to the state of despair. The self in demonic despair is a self who clings to his or her despair. It is a self who is not, on any account, willing to let go of the despair; a self who would rather be *right* than be *redeemed*; a self who does not want to seek help even if that means living through "all the agonies of hell."[6] Suffice to say that this demonic logic is certainly not entirely alien to Houellebecq's protagonists.

In the beginning of *Sickness unto Death*, Kierkegaard writes that, normally, *to be able to be* this or that does not have the same status as *to be* this or that. Reality or actuality (*Virkelighed*) is on a higher level than possibility (*Mulighed*). For this reason, he states that "being is related to the ability to be as an ascent."[7] With despair the situation is completely different: "With respect to despair, however, to be is like a descent when compared with being able to be; the descent is infinitely low as the excellence of possibility is high."[8] To be is thus related to the ability to be as *a fall*. "Infinite as is the advantage of the possibility," Kierkegaard notes with stunning clarity, "just so great is the measure of the fall."[9] This means that in the case of despair possibility stands above actuality. The self in despair experiences a *fall* from the self that could be to the self that is or, alternatively, a fall from the future to the present. If anxiety, as Kierkegaard defines it, is to be compared with the feeling of vertigo or dizziness one experiences when staring *down* into the abyss of existence, into the void of freedom, the nothingness of being, then despair may be imagined as the feeling of standing or lying down in that abysmal hole while looking *up*.

This peculiar relationship between up and down, between what is possible and what is necessary, between present and future, is in any case what defines despair according to Kierkegaard, and it is also what defines the paradigmatic scene in *Whatever*. "It's not that I feel tremendously low, it's rather that the world around me appears high," the narrator explains.[10] But rather than emphasizing the mis-relation between a present/actual and future/possible self – that is, a mis-relation within the self – as Kierkegaard tends to do, Houellebecq is much more interested in the mis-relation – or desynchronization to use Thomas Fuchs' concept – between self and world. Another obvious difference: The main character in *Whatever* is not (just) in despair, he is depressed.[11] Though he mocks the psychiatrist and the whole realm of psychiatry, not to mention psychology – for example, taking great pains to describe the fancy watch ("fawn leather strap, rectangular gold-plated face") that the psychiatrist wears and repeatedly glances at before delivering his diagnosis in the most routine like manner – and though the narrator, as well as the novel as a whole, is clearly not interested in the *diagnosis* or the *name* of depression, the *reality* of depression is examined to the point of exhaustion.

Depressive realism?

Does this warrant or justify a reading of Houellebecq as a depressive realist, not only in the sense that he captures the reality of depressive suffering, but also that he captures the reality from a depressive perspective?

In itself, the depression to be found in Houellebecq seems to constitute a negative optical system, a bleak and pessimistic world-view. In the book Ghosts of My Life, to which I referred earlier, Mark Fisher writes that "[d]epression is, after all and above all, a theory about the world, about life [...] Depression is not sadness, not even a state of mind, it is a (neuro)philosophical (dis)position."[12] A certain pessimism, perhaps even cynicism or nihilism, appears to be at work here. It is no coincidence that the first book Houellebecq ever wrote and published was a monograph on the American horror fiction writer H. P. Lovecraft, *H.P. Lovecraft. Against the World, Against Life* (1991). The title of the book says it all, but in case that is not enough, one could content oneself with consulting the following emphatic line from Lovecraft's story "Facts Concerning the Late Arthur Jermyn and His Family," also quoted by Houellebecq: "Life is a hideous thing, and from the background behind what we know of it peer daemoniacal hints of truth which make it sometimes a thousandfold more hideous."[13]

Of course, Houellebecq has also read Pascal and Schopenhauer, compulsory reading for any proper pessimist. But Lovecraft was the true love: Here Houellebecq has found an endless source of inspiration with regards to the pessimistic view of the world, the deep disgust with society and the endless rants against what Lovecraft called *smirking optimism* in the essay "Supernatural horror in literature." As the narrator of *Whatever* broadcasts: "I don't like this world. I definitely do not like it. The society in which I live disgusts me; advertising sickens me; computers make me puke."[14]

There is, however, something suspicious – treacherous even – about these prototypical Houellebecqian statements. They testify to the danger of the depressive position, the risk of being seduced by the wisdom and clarity that seem to emanate from it: A seduction that goes not only in the direction of the one who listens to or reads the depressive's tirades, but also concerns the depressed person himself. Again, Mark Fisher describes this very well: "The depressive is always confident of one thing: that he is without illusion [...] Depressive ontology is dangerously seductive because, as the zombie twin of a certain philosophical wisdom, it is half true."[15] Or as Jonathan Franzen – who has also written perceptively about his colleague and friend David Foster Wallace – writes in the essay "Why Bother?": "Depression presents itself as a realism regarding the rottenness of the world in general and the rottenness of your life in particular. But the realism is merely a mask for depression's actual essence, which is an overwhelming estrangement from humanity."[16] In that sense, what presents itself as a total lack of illusions may in fact be the ultimate illusion; what appears as a certain realism about the world, an objective assessment, can very well be a psychological defense mechanism as well, a routine to fall back on, a mask to hide behind.

Such accusations would not be totally unwarranted in the case of Houellebecq, but I would like to question the assumption that Houellebecq is such a primitive writer – or so caught up in demonic despair – that he identifies his personal collapse with the collapse of the world. There are, in other words, enough reasons to be wary of the hypothesis of depressive realism, which – as mentioned earlier – holds that depressed people have a more accurate and realistic assessment of the world than non-depressed people do; that they have, in the words of Freud, "a keener eye for the truth than others who are not melancholic."[17] In the scholarship on Houellebecq, though, this kind of thinking has remained quite influential, leading to the widespread perception that his depressed protagonists – or Houellebecq as the depressed author – are in possession of a special knowledge about the society and world they live in.[18] Thus, Houellebecqian sentences about the horror of the modern world – society is disgusting, work is meaningless, life is useless – are taken at face value, as plain truths about the world; as insights that even sociology must envy. My point here is that there is no guarantee that the statements, which issue from the depressive position, rise above the level of banality. In fact, a lot of the sentences do not transgress standard pessimist phrases or clichés. In addition to this problem of *banality*, there is a problem of *inconsistency* in Houellebecq's work and world. At one moment, the individual is taken to be a pure expression of social and historical processes, only to be regarded within the framework of a stern biological determinism or a Lovecraftian cosmology the next. This is made even clearer if we turn to Houellebecq's other novels: Suddenly the traumatic childhood of Bruno in *Atomised* is, for example, presented as the cause of his adult misery, while psychology is denounced in other places as the most ridiculous science of all.

There is a general consideration I would like to interpolate here, namely that it is important not to surrender too quickly to the captivating concept of depressive realism: One might end up in the cul-de-sac of causality, in the labyrinth of etiological explanations. It should be remembered that Houellebecq is not a psychologist, but he is not a sociologist either, nor an economist for that matter (Bernard Maris has written a whole book called *Houellebecq. Economiste* (2014)). Despite what most people seem to believe, Houellebecq is, first and last, a writer, who is surely allowed his fair share of (self-)contradictions. More explicitly, he is a writer who deals with depression, but only in the sense that his literature is a construction and exploration of depressive symptoms. It is more a symptomatology than an etiology. Or to put it another way: What is noteworthy about Houellebecq's account of the political anatomy of depression is not so much the criticism of society that he consistently performs and advances, as the depressive position *from which* this criticism is raised. At times the statements appear banal but the toneless voice *with which* these statements is delivered is itself far from banal.

This does not mean that realism cannot be found in the works of Houellebecq, but that the realism is located elsewhere, in what I would call *a symptomatological realism* rather than a depressive realism. As for *Whatever*, this truly self-aware debut novel is unafraid of laying bare its own endeavor. No more psychological realism, the novel declares at the very beginning, though this is not to be taken as a rejection of realism *per se*: "All that accumulation of realistic detail, with clearly differentiated characters hogging the limelight has always seemed pure bullshit to me [...] Might as well watch lobsters marching up the side of an aquarium."[19] In direct continuity with this preliminary design of a new poetics, a later passage reads:

> This progressive effacement of human relationships is not without certain problems for the novel. How, in point of fact, would one handle the narration of those unbridled passions, stretching over many years, and at times making their effect felt on several generations? We're a long way from *Wuthering Heights*, to say the least. The novel form is not conceived for depicting indifference or nothingness; a flatter, more terse, and dreary discourse would need to be invented.[20]

This is, in fact, what Houellebecq preaches and practices, not only in *Whatever*, but in his whole *oeuvre*, and the reason he is often accused of being a fundamentally bad writer. His syntax is too simple, his style too uninspired, people claim. Just look, for example, at the beginning of *Whatever*: "Friday evening I was invited to a party at a colleague from work's house. There were thirty-odd of us, all middle management aged between twenty-five and forty."[21] Sure enough, a chain of main clauses seems to drag themselves – and the reader – along. There is a complete lack of affective vibration in the narrator's voice. The tonal register is flat, the intonation without any ring, the language as a whole appears empty and inanimate. These are indeed typical traits of any Houellebecq novel, but that is exactly the point: The invention of "a flatter, more terse and dreary discourse." What we have here is "a kind of limp *déjà dit*," as Victoria Best and Martin Crowley correctly point out: "we all know everything already (including, of course, the fact that we all know everything already…)."[22] The stylistic effect – or rather affect – is the feeling of exhaustion at having said it all before, of having to repeat oneself over and over again. It is, I would claim, a symptomatic discourse, a discourse symptomatic of depression. But Houellebecq's symptomatology goes deeper than that.

On one level, some of Houellebecq's sci-fi scenarios of the future in his other books can be read as being so rudimentary that it is hard not to view them as signs of a collapsed imagination. The very construction of works like *Atomised* and *The Possibility of an Island* seems to be a symptom of an artistic imagination that cannot escape the depressive condition of pure uncreativity (Ben Jeffery has articulated the original idea that "Houellebecq's books are works of the imagination against the imagination. They hate themselves."[23]). On another level, the symptomatology pertains to the scope of the characters' imagination – or lack of it. When, for example, Daniel – the main character in *The Possibility of an Island* – finds a young girlfriend and one of the primary differences between the two characters manifests in their different conceptions of capitalism: "Capitalism was for her [Esther] a natural habitat, in which she moved with the grace that characterized all the actions in her life; to strike in protest of planned redundancies would have seemed to her as absurd as striking against the weather getting colder, or the invasion of North Africa by crickets."[24] Capitalism is Esther's natural habitat, which makes it difficult for her to imagine the end of capitalism, let alone an alternative to it. In a talk given at The Royal Danish Academy of Fine Arts in February 2014 under the title "On some of the affects of capitalism," Bruno Latour addressed this relationship between nature and society, between earth and the capitalist economy, between first nature and second nature, between "binding necessities" and "boundless possibilities." Latour's point was that the relationship has been turned upside down so that today it is nature and the natural laws that appear as a field of contingency and subject to change, whereas capitalism has been transformed into a kind of first nature that seems as unalterable as the laws of nature used to be: "It is the Earth that is undergoing subversion at a dizzying pace and the Economy – that is, second nature – that still runs like clockwork."[25] As for Esther in *The Possibility of an Island*, this constitutes no problem at all, causing no despairing or depressive feelings, since all she has ever known is the capitalist clockwork. It is totally different for Daniel and all the other (male) narrators and protagonists of Houellebecq's books; every single one *has* known some moment of happiness uncorrupted by capitalism, a brief period of pure love, or something like that. This explains the occasionally nostalgic or even sentimental tone of the narrators: An awareness of things that have been, or could have been, or could be different. Against such awareness, the present state of things, including the capitalist clockwork, stands out like an abysmal and claustrophobic dungeon. This contrast – foreign to Esther and the people of her generation – is similar to a Kierkegaardian dialectic between necessity and possibility: If you have not had an experience of being *up there*, or of aspiring to some possible other state floating above your head, it is difficult to feel *down*. Which brings me back to *Whatever*.

It is two in the afternoon

As already mentioned, at the end of the novel the narrator and main protagonist is diagnosed with depression and hospitalized. After being discharged, he travels to Saint-Cirgues-en-Montagne, specifically the Forest of Mazan. At this point in time he realizes that his horizon of action has been severely limited: "My margin of manoeuvre in life has become singularly restricted. I still envisage a number of possibilities, but they only vary in points of detail."[26] Here the possible has finally given way to the impossible. In a rather crude sense: Necessity wins. The problem is not that he cannot choose between this or that possibility, but that he cannot choose choice itself. Choice as such has disappeared; the possibility of possibility has evaporated from the horizon. As Kierkegaard writes in part II of *Either/Or*, "action is essentially future tense," adding a few pages later: "As truly, then, as there is a time to come, so truly there is an Either/Or."[27] But to the depressive narrator there is precisely no "time to come" and *eo ipso* no Either/Or. There is no longer any future *whatsoever*.

And so, as the novel closes, he goes deeper into the woods: "I am at the heart of the abyss. I feel my skin again as a frontier, and the external world as a crushing weight. The impression of separation is total; from now on I am imprisoned within myself. It will not take place, the sublime fusion; the goal of life is missed. It is two in the afternoon."[28] Here it is imperative to pay attention to indications of time, mention of specific dates, and, not least, use of grammatical tenses. It is evident that the novel has a partiality for bringing the reader's attention to seemingly insignificant times of day, such as the description of a peculiar incident when the protagonist witnesses another man's sudden death that ends with the words: "All in a day's work. It was six-twenty."[29] It is six-twenty, it is two in the afternoon. The male protagonists always know exactly what time it is. Crucially, these temporal designations can be understood as expressions of what Thomas Fuchs calls the explicit temporality of depression: A desynchronization, a loss of the individual's familiarity with his surroundings and the world. Unquestionably, this is where Michel finds himself at the end of *Whatever*: In a situation within which time has become mercilessly explicit.

The final sequence of *Whatever* performs this gradual explicitation of time, as attention is increasingly turned toward the passing of time *itself*, culminating, as previously noted, in the final phrase: "It is two in the afternoon." But time does not simply become explicit; it acquires, concurrently, a certain diabolical quality. The diabolical horror is not that things end, but that they do not and cannot end. Time has become not dead, but undead. As Kierkegaard writes in *Sickness unto Death*: "the torment of despair is precisely this inability to die. [...] Thus to be sick *unto* death is to be unable to die, yet not as if there were hope of life; no, the hopelessness is that there is not even the ultimate hope, death."[30] This may explain and account for the present tense of the ultimate statement: It *is* two in the afternoon. Up to this point, the novel has mainly operated in the past tense, though occasionally and sporadically it has shifted to the present tense. However, toward the end, particularly in the final section, "Saint-Cirgues-en-Montagne," the use of the present tense is intensified, bearing witness, perhaps, to an endless now, a suffering without end. In this sense, the final designation of time may be a form of period, but the very present tense of the sentence seems to hold the situation open, extending the depressive's anguish ad infinitum.

Scene 2. "A permanent state of war" (*Atomised*)

December 31st 1999 fell on a Friday. In the clinic at Verrières-le-Buisson, where Bruno would spend the rest of his life, there was a small party for the patients and the care staff. They drank champagne and ate paprika-flavoured crisps. Later that evening Bruno danced with one of the nurses. He wasn't unhappy; the medication was working, he no longer had any feelings of desire. He enjoyed the afternoon snack, and watching game shows on television with the others before the evening meal. He expected nothing, now, of the progression of days, and the last night of the second millennium was a pleasant one for him.

In cemeteries all across the world, the recently deceased continued to rot in their graves, slowly becoming skeletons.

Michel spent the evening at home. He was too isolated to hear the noise of the party in the village. Many times, warm and peaceful images of Annabelle flitted across his memory, and images too of his grandmother.

He remembered that when he was 13 or 14 he used to buy flashlights, and small mechanical objects which he liked to take apart and put together again endlessly. And he remembered an aeroplane with a motor which his grandmother had given him, which he had never succeeded in flying. It was a beautiful plane, painted in camouflage; in the end, it stayed in its box. Through the slow drift of his consciousness, certain things seemed to characterize his life. There were people and thoughts. Thoughts occupy no space; people occupy a portion of space; they can be seen. Their images form on the lens, pass through the choroid and strike the retina. Alone in the empty house, Michel watched his modest parade of memories. Throughout the evening, a single conviction slowly filled his mind: soon he would be able to get back to work.

All across the surface of the globe, a weary, exhausted humanity, filled with self-doubt and uncertain of its history, prepared itself as best as it could to enter a new millennium.[31]

What do depressives dream of? And what kind of dream – or nightmare – is the so-called Y2K? What kind of historical time is revealed through this New Year's Eve of 1999 in Michel Houellebecq's novel *Atomised* (1998)? Is it History – with a capital H – that comes to an end here? Is what we are dealing with, in that case, nothing but a confirmation of the depressive's premonition and longing: That everything is finally over? Or is it, rather, a question of the verification of the depressive's ultimate fear: That things in fact do *not* come to an end? Does the millennial change bear witness to a crisis in time, an un-ecstatic and end-less time: an end without end? Is this what the countdown is all about? A countdown to zero and then what? Death? Or infinity? Immortality? These are the questions, and hidden behind them is a question of the political economy, more specifically: May 1968 and neoliberal competition.

Bruno and Michel

What a lovely pair they make, Michel and Bruno, the two half-brothers and protagonists of *Atomised*, celebrating New Year separately in the scene above. On the whole, the story is narrated in the third-person from somewhere in the future; it is set in the year 2029 at least, probably further ahead in time, since in the narrator's present almost every living creature is a clone and the last representatives of humanity are dying. *Atomised* is, in a certain sense, designed as an obituary to "a weary exhausted" humankind. The epilogue finishes with the sentence: "This book is dedicated to mankind."[32] The mankind which – thank God? – no longer is. From the futural perspective of the book, the human is already *a thing of the past*. This is the temporal frame of the story: We are in the future looking back to the past, which is our present. And the loss of that present is not exactly something to mourn.

Michel Djerzinski – a world-renowned molecular biologist – and Bruno Clément – a provincial high school teacher – are totally different but equally depressed. Leading a life governed by sexual impulses, Bruno feels, from a very early age, the competition that pervades not only the sphere of economy, but the sphere of sexuality as well: the expanded field of battle as it were. Pain, suffering and premature ejaculation characterize his life, with the exception of the occasional stay at the 1968 hippy-ish place "Lieu du Changement" – holiday resort and swinger club in one – where Bruno meets Christiane and experiences brief moments of intense happiness, as the novel is fond of formulating it. But Christiane suffers an injury that leaves her disabled and subsequently commits suicide. As a result, Bruno turns to drinking, becomes increasingly aggressive and depressive, until he finally breaks down after trying to seduce an Arab girl from the high school class that he teaches. He is then put in a psychiatric clinic; a "depressed teacher, possibly suicidal," in the laconic words of the novel.[33] It is here that we meet Bruno in the scene above, in a psychiatric hospital on New Year's Eve: "He wasn't unhappy; the medication was working, he no longer had any feelings of desire." This state of medicalized numbness – no feelings of desire, no expectations – is the closest Bruno comes to happiness. Or, to be more precise, the questions of happiness and unhappiness no longer make any sense: He is beyond both. Here, a lack of expectations, hopes and dreams are presented not as a cause or even as a symptom of depression, but rather as a solution to the state of depression. The problem with Bruno is not that he does not expect anything, but that he was previously expecting too much. This is what has induced so much misery. That problem has now been solved and the new millennium can come as it may. If there is no hope, there can be no despair either. On various occasions, Bruno is described as a thoroughly typical individual, which conversely makes it hard to conceive of him as an individual. He is typical because he continues to play a game that he cannot win; because the sexual economy of the West is not meant for people like him; because he, as he himself sadly declares, "is completely dependent" on a society in which he plays "no useful role."[34] He is ultimately all too human.

Michel, on the other hand, is the atypical individual; highly, almost frighteningly intelligent, and not really a human being at all. Never exhibiting any real emotions – "the world of human emotions was not his field" – he leads "a purely intellectual existence."[35] No events or incidents are able to move or touch him, which is why Bruno at one point tells Michel that Michel is not human. As described in the scene under scrutiny here: "[C]ertain things seemed to characterize his life. There were people and thoughts." What a life: People and thoughts! Even his high school sweetheart Annabel – who is otherwise capable of making any boy or man swoon – does not rouse his desire. But is it the case that Michel does not feel anything, or would it be more accurate to say that what he is experiencing is the feeling of not feeling anything? Regardless, at the end of the novel Michel travels to Ireland, tellingly described as "the westernmost point of Europe, the very edge of the Western world."[36] In the epilogue we are told – from a future point of view and thus in the past tense – of Michel's last days in the ancient year of 2009, before he left, disappeared, or committed suicide, as is believed: One day, he apparently walked out into the ocean and disappeared.

Michel is thus everything that Bruno is not, and vice versa. They are, in the most classical manner, each other's mirror images. Bruno is utterly at the mercy of his feelings; Michel is perfectly numb and inclined to cool abstraction. Bruno is almost addicted to sex; Michel seems completely uninterested in erotic adventures. Bruno is suffering from a kind of hedonia, Michel from anhedonia.[37] But both become depressed. Both become inhuman, but from opposite directions.

Neoliberal competition and May '68 (the horror, the horror)

In *Atomised*, the primary problem articulated and criticized *through* the experience of depression is the event and aftermath of May '68. Bruno and Michel's mother, Janine, is the paradigmatic embodiment of everything that this event stood and continues to stand for: A general progressiveness, a fundamental emancipation of desire, and a stubborn quest for an autonomous life, not to mention mind-expanding drugs. According to the novel, '68 may very well have been perceived as "a communist utopia," a collective project, but in reality it was just "another stage in the rise of the individual."[38] In fact, Bruno thinks that there is an intimate connection between this individualism, the narcissistic pursuit of pleasure, and physical violence: "In a sense, the serial killers of the 1990s were the spiritual children of the hippies of the Sixties [...] From this point of view, Charles Manson was not some monstrous aberration in the hippie movement, but its logical conclusion."[39]

There is no doubt that every statement that Bruno tosses off must be interpreted with certain reservations considering his consumption of alcohol, his psychic condition and his general outlook described by the narrator as "a cynical, hard-bitten, typically masculine view of life,"[40] which says quite a lot. While many of Bruno's tirades are tiresome to listen to, the same can be said of many of the novel's misogynistic comments, the bashing of feminism, the Islamophobic remarks and so on. That said, the critique of '68 must be taken seriously, because it is a – if not *the* – constant in Houellebecq's body of work. In *Atomised* the harsh view of May '68 culminates in a scene during the summer of 1974 – recounted by Bruno to his psychiatrist – when a young Bruno walks into his mother's bedroom, where she is asleep beside one of her countless lovers, pulls off the sheet, kneels down and looks directly up into her vagina. This is not just a childish fantasy, this is indeed the night of the world, May '68.

The fundamental principle, or ideological imperative, that is at work and subject to criticism in *Atomised* – as in all of Houellebecq's other novels for that matter – is *competition* (part two of *Platform* is, for example, called simply "Competitive Advantage"). This is integral to the analysis of '68 as the background for the "general mood of depression" in "the last years of Western civilization."[41] Here, the history of '68 and the history of neoliberalism become one in the world and work of Houellebecq.[42]

As Michel Foucault detailed in the series of lectures published as *The Birth of Biopolitics*, in neoliberalism "Homo Economicus is an entrepreneur, an entrepreneur of himself."[43] Within the neoliberal theory of *human capital* – Gary Becker's book *Human Capital* was published in 1964 and the concept quickly became a standard reference within neoliberalism, although the concept had existed and flourished for some years before that – the human is quite simply viewed as capital, or as an investor whose primary (re)source of investment, whose fundamental form of capital, is him or herself. Here, competition is not just something that is nourished and thrives in the market economy, or within the institutional framework of the so-called competition state. Rather it is as if competition has become an ontological or anthropological reality. As Margaret Thatcher once said: "Economics are the method; the object is to change the heart and soul."

For Houellebecq, the primary consequence of the neoliberal economy that has emerged and developed in the wake of May '68 is thus the creation of a world in which competition makes itself felt at any time and in any location. According to his books, neoliberalism is all about extending or expanding the zone of struggle. It goes without saying that, if vacations and leisure time have also become a question of self-realization, there will be an element of competition there too. This is what his books show: That the tentacles of competition do not only reach into the working sphere but into life as such, into the very being and soul of each individual, just as Thatcher understood and recommended. Of special relevance is the way in which Houellebecq's continuous and concentrated thematization of work is less about a change in *the work* than about a change of *the worker* and his or her personality. It is in this sense that one must read the statement in *Platform,* that capitalism is a permanent state of war.[44]

Science: Our last, great adventure

In principle, there are only two responses to this situation, to this permanent state of war with no external limits and no outside. As Carole Sweeney observes: "If there is no outside, no space of opposition, then our only options, Houellebecq suggests, are either hedonistic participation or an ascetic retreat."[45] Bruno and Michel are the very obvious incarnations of "hedonistic participation" and "ascetic retreat," respectively. The truly devastating insight is that it does not really matter which you choose, both paths lead to the same door of depression as the New Year's Eve of 1999 testifies to. An evening traditionally constituting an occasion for anticipation, expectation, hope, a new beginning, a rite of passage into the future, has here degenerated into a passage to nothing.

Of course the Millennium Bug, as it was known, now appears deeply dated and rather ridiculous, and yet something significant takes place in *Atomised.* Or rather, something significant does *not* take place. In the novel, in this particular scene, it is as if the year 2000 does not really happen. How are we to understand this?

I think that Jean Baudrillard's *The Vital Illusion* can be of some help here. In the book, he advances precisely the idea that the year 2000 would not take place: "[B]ecause the history of this century had already come to an end, because we are remaking it interminably and because, therefore, metaphorically speaking, we shall never pass on, into the future."[46] Baudrillard calls this phenomenon "a reversal of our modern relation to time" in the sense that:

> time is no longer counted progressively, by addition, starting from an origin – but by subtraction, starting from the end. This is what happens with rocket launches and time bombs. And that end is no longer the symbolic endpoint of a history but the mark of a zero sum, of a potential exhaustion. Time is viewed from a perspective of entropy – the exhausting of all possibilities – the perspective of a counting down...to infinity.[47]

This historical relation to history, this specific temporal experience, is emphasized by Houellebecq in the New Year's Eve scene in *Atomised*: The sense that there is no future and nothing to look forward to, since all possibilities have been exhausted in advance; the sense that history is already over and humanity no longer exists. When the end – the year 2000 – finally arrives a strange sensation of *déjà vu* surfaces. The brothers may be as different as night and day but in the end their problem is the same: A problem of the end. As Baudrillard writes: "Our millenarianism – for we have reached, all the same, a millenarian deadline – is *a millenarianism with no tomorrow*."[48]

It is here that the dreams of cloning and of immortality come into play. It may seem paradoxical, for who in his or her right mind would want to extend a miserable life into the infinite? (One of the first phrases of *The Possibility of an Island* reads: Who, among you, deserves eternal life? Yet the question is, rather: Who among you wants eternal life?) But the point is, as Baudrillard is once again able to clarify, that "[i]n cloning – this collective fantasy of a return to a nonindividuated existence and a destiny of undifferentiated life, this temptation to return to an indifferent immortality – we see the very form of a repentance of the living toward the unliving."[49] This fantasy or temptation betrays a certain Freudian death-drive, which is precisely not a desire to die, but a desire to keep on living in a kind of undead or zombie-like state, where every possible form of individuation, sexualization and differentiation has been eliminated, not to mention desire itself. "This may well be the story of a deliberate project to put an end to the genetic game of difference, to stop the divagations of the living," Baudrillard writes in *The Vital Illussion*, before posing the somewhat rhetorical question: "Aren't we actually sick of sex, of difference, of emancipation, of culture?"[50]

Houellebecq's answer is an affirmative and resounding yes. This is indeed what his novels and characters are sick of and why the event of 1968, and everything it stands for and has led to, is portrayed as the paramount culprit. This is also the reason that the character of Michel is a scientist in molecular biology in *Atomised*. His research focuses on developing the scientific preconditions for the perfect reproduction. His epoch-making scientific discovery, when he returns to work after the New Year's Eve of 1999, is that every cell can be copied, infinitely and perfectly. Forget about the genetic cloning of sheep and cows; what must be cloned are human beings themselves. This is Michel's radical proposal: "[t]hat humanity must disappear, that humanity would give way to a new species which was asexual and immortal, a species which had outgrown individuality, individuation, and progress."[51] The goal is to eliminate the differentiation and individuation that underlie the principle of competition. The goal is to achieve a world without desire, without feelings, without happiness and thus also without unhappiness: a blissful numbness, or, in the words of Baudrillard, "an indifferent immortality." The goal is to arrive at a stage where beings are no longer "sexed, differentiated, and mortal."[52] It is to accomplish an exit from history, which is an exit from humanity, an exit from being human. This is the revenge, the only solution to the problem of a depressed and exhausted humanity.

It is clear within the imaginary of *Atomised* that science and technology are the only means through which this fantasy can be realized. Science is indeed "our last adventure, our last great narrative, the bearer of dreams as well as nightmares, and it alone is capable of combining poetry, action and utopia."[53] Or as Bruno Latour suggests: Science is politics by other means. Interestingly, this notion of genetic manipulation, of a "revolutionary" transformation of the self, is a direct continuation of the neoliberal idea of the self as human capital which, as Philip Mirowski has convincingly argued, is not unrelated to the experiments with the self that took place in the drug culture of the 1960s and the events preceding, constituting and following May '68. Foucault made this connection explicitly, albeit from a slightly different perspective: "The malleability of the self presumed by the theory of human capital investment will extend down to the most basic corporal level, which will eventually mean investment in genetic manipulation."[54] Technological alteration, customization and optimization of the self are absolutely integral to the neoliberal mindset. As Mirowski writes: "The ultimate goal of genetics is therefore a DNA upgrade: the ability to freely alter yourself at will at the ribonucleic level [...] *This is the true terminus of the neoliberal self.*"[55]

In a sense Houellebecq takes this at face value, and even takes it one step further: Within the horizon of his novel, the ambition is not to improve the self but to leave the self – as we know it – behind. The "first or final point of resistance" does not consist in "the relation of self to self" as it does for Foucault.[56] Nor is a pharmacological neuroenhancement anywhere near radical enough, though Bruno is temporarily relieved of his misery in the scene above: "He wasn't unhappy; the medication was working, he no longer had any feelings of desire." The solution in the works of Houellebecq – if there is such a thing as a solution; not at all a rhetorical question – is neither ethical nor chemical, but ontological or technological. It is the very biological and ontological reality of the human that must be manipulated. In Houellebecq, being human is not impossible; it is simply unbearable...

But is a technological posthumanity or an artificial neohumanity a real solution? Is it really the case that "the solution to every problem – whether psychological, sociological or more broadly human – could only be a technical solution" and that "THE REVOLUTION WILL NOT BE MENTAL, BUT GENETIC" as it is stated toward the end of *Atomised*?[57] Is that the true terminus of the twin trajectories of neoliberalism and May '68? Is this the only way to enter the new millennium, or is the dream of cloning and immortality actually more like a depressive dream, a symptom of a depressive imagination?

Scene 3. The possibility of not being depressed? (*The possibility of an island*)

The sight before me was almost the same in all directions; but I knew that to the southwest, once the fault had been crossed, from the heights of Leganes or maybe Fuenlabrada, I was going to have to make my way across the Great Gray Space. Estremadura and Portugal had disappeared as differentiated places. The succession of nuclear explosions, of tidal waves, of cyclones that had battered this geographical zone for several centuries had ended up completely flattening its surface and transforming it into one vast sloping place, of weak declivity, which appeared in satellite photos as uniformly composed of pulverulent ashes of a very light gray color. This sloping place continued for about two and a half thousand kilometers before opening out upon a little-known region of the world, whose sky was almost continually saturated with light clouds and vapors, situated on the site of the former Canary Islands.[58]

The "I" of this passage is Daniel25: A clone, replicant and so-called *neohuman*. He is a descendent of Daniel1, whom we meet and follow in the first two-thirds of the novel *The Possibility of an Island*. Daniel1 is another prototypical Houellebecqian protagonist, thoroughly depressive in the world of today. A comedian, he has staged controversial shows such as *We Prefer the Palestinian Orgy Sluts* and the film *Munch of My Gaza Strip (My Huge Jewish Settler)*, which has earned him all the fame and money in the world, but, unsurprisingly, no happiness. He has a wife but after she leaves him he finds himself on the verge of joining a sect called the Elohimites (modulated on the Raëlian movement). It is a big joke – the prophet and leader of the sect wears a t-shirt with the text "lick my balls" – and yet the religion of the Elohimites achieves world hegemony, because the sect manages to develop the technology of cloning, making the dream of becoming immortal a reality. In the words of one critic, nicely summarizing the rest of Daniel1's life, Daniel ends up "leaving DNA in deep freeze before writing his life story and committing suicide. He rematerializes eons later as Daniel2, then 3 through 25." *The Possibility of an Island* thus makes manifest a fictional realization of the technical solution to the problem of a depressed and weary humanity proposed at the end of *Atomised* (for me these two books thus form a kind of duology). To a great extent, the future world presented in the former begins where the latter breaks off. The key to grasping whether a technological posthumanity or an artificial neohumanity is a real solution or not is Daniel25.

Daniel25 and a Lovecraftian landscape of clinical depression

Daniel25 lives in a world many, many years into the distant future; a post-apocalyptic world transformed and destroyed by climate change, nuclear bombs, tidal waves, cyclones and other catastrophes. It is a world no longer dependent upon sexual and biological reproduction because it is possible to "bypass the embryogenesis stage and directly manufacture adult individuals."[59] This only requires the transfer of DNA, as well as memory and personality through some so-called life stories, from one generation to the next, which is what Daniel1 has done while with the Elohimites and thus achieved eternal life. In this world, all needs are reduced to an absolute minimum: Interpersonal relations, including masturbation, take place via the internet, and food is ingested by means of a photosynthetic system, which makes neohumans capable of surviving on small amounts of water and a few minerals. The result is, in the words of the novel, "nothing less than a new species and even, strictly speaking, a new kingdom."[60] The kingdom of no desire, as it were.

In *The Possibility of an Island*, this new kingdom is intended as a kind of utopia; the suffering of being and the competition between beings have been eliminated, in the sense that money and sex have been done away with. What exists is a "freedom of indifference," an "obvious neutrality of the real." There are no plans, no becoming, no difference, no change. In the words of Daniel25: "I had attained innocence, in an absolute and nonconflictual state, I no longer had any plan, nor any objective, and my individuality dissolved into an indefinite series of days; I was happy."[61] A blissful state of sterile and hermit-like happiness. But, of course, this is not entirely true. As Daniel25 also admits: "Happiness should have come [...] but happiness had not come."[62]

An increasing and thoroughly human dissatisfaction with life in the new kingdom finds its way into the novel and the mind of Daniel25, up to the point where, in the last part of the book, he embarks upon a journey in order to experience something new. In an act combining hope and despair, he leaves his isolated and excluded reservation – outside which the last remains of the old humanity rummages around – and heads for what were formerly known as the Canary Islands. What Daniel25 confronts and experiences here is a deeply Lovecraftian world, reminiscent of the "glacial void of 700 miles" chillingly described in Lovecraft's *At the Mountains of Madness*.[63] As Charles Baxter has argued in an article in *The New York Review of Books*, what Lovecraft was truly writing about was the horror of clinical depression: "In some sense Lovecraft does not write about 'horrors' at all but about the worst kinds of clinical depression, the feeling that one is dead but not dead enough to achieve real rest. Nothing gives pleasure, nor can any form of pleasure be imagined."[64]

Indeed, it is the mountains of madness or the glacial void of depression that meet Daniel25 at the end of his journey. In the quoted passage from *The Possibility of an Island*, the glacial void is a sloping plane of ash and salt, continuing for about "two and a half thousand kilometers before opening out upon a little-known region of the world."[65] Is it possible to conceive of this landscape as anything other than a landscape of clinical depression? As is well known, depression is not merely an economic or a psychiatric/psychological category; it is also a geological appellation for a land-form sunk below the level of the surrounding area. This seems to be what Houellebecq is depicting in the scene in question. In a sense, it is no longer possible to distinguish the mental and material catastrophe, as if the internal and external landscapes melt into each other, in so far as the external is more an extension than an expression of the internal. It is not a metaphor; the landscape functions more as a literalization of metaphors usually employed to describe a pathological state of depression. Depression is often described as a feeling of gliding or sinking, of losing your footing and of the ground disappearing from under you, or, alternatively, as a sensation that everything is frozen, dried up. Here, this feeling is concretized, made literal. Once again the real horror is that of not even being able to die; of experiencing "that one is dead but not dead enough to achieve real rest."

"The future was empty"

The models of technology and science in the novels of *Atomised* and *The Possibility of an Island* do not lead anywhere but to an affirmation of the *status quo*; to an infinitization of the depressive condition. This is made clear through a paradoxical twofold relation between present and future that is operative in the novels.

First, the future is already present, it is already here. In *Atomised,* an unlimited, indefinite stasis is not something awaiting us, but something happening right now, or that has even already happened. The annihilation of humanity *is* a reality; the dream – or the nightmare – *has* already manifested itself, not least as far as Michel– whose life can be perceived as a paradigmatic example of the "*obvious* neutrality of the real" that the future was supposed to bring about in *The Possibility of an Island*[66] – is concerned. To Michel, sex and money do not matter and common human emotions are not available to him. He is already living as a cyborg or a clone. This is what the very first scene of *Atomised* shows: Human communication and interaction is impossible. After his own farewell reception at work, which opens the novel, Michel finds himself standing in the parking lot with a female colleague: They try to politely and appropriately take leave of one another, but the exchange is excruciatingly awkward. In a sense, this small scene summons the end of the human civilization as we know it. When Michel is driving home, he feels as though he is in a sci-fi-movie, as if he is "the last man on earth after every other living thing had been wiped out. A post-apocalyptic wasteland."[67] The future, then, is already present, or the human present is already inhuman.

Secondly, the future world presented in *The Possibility of an Island*, beginning where *Atomised* ends, is only an extension and continuation of the present. What *could be* is reduced to what *is*. The techno-scientific solution to the problems of the Western world and the therapeutic overcoming of depression solve nothing. There is no qualitative difference between then and now. The post-human or neohuman is still all too human. Daniel25 cannot help but hope or despair, which in the end almost amounts to one and the same thing. His only source of dialog, Marie23 – who incites his journey of rebellion – is described precisely as being still all too human. In that sense, the future is just like the present, or the inhuman future is always too human.

There is, in other words, no rupture or discontinuity between the present and the future in the universe of Houellebecq. This is what leads up to and explains the ending of *The Possibility of an Island*:

I had perhaps sixty years left to live; more than twenty thousand days that would be identical [...] Happiness was not a possible horizon. The world had betrayed. My body belonged to me for only a brief lapse of time; I would never reach the goal I had been set. The future was empty; it was the mountain. My dreams were populated with emotional presences. I was, I was no longer. Life was real.[68]

Moments before he ostensibly dies, Daniel25 is faced with an endless horizon, a flat world in every respect, or rather a slightly sloping surface, a small yet steady inclination, and a minimal but inevitable fall into nothing. But also: a mountain. Again, the topography is striking, exhibiting a down and an up. Equally, if we pay close attention to the grammatical tense, we cannot help but notice the use of the past tense in this final section – the epilogue – of the novel, whereas the tense has shifted back and forth between past and present until that point. It is not the case that the future *is* empty: From the final displaced and advanced point of narration the future *was* empty ("Le future était vide"). From this point and perspective, the future is something that *was*; a thing of the past. To paraphrase the writer Jaris-Karl Huysmans, who plays a central part in *Submission*: The future has had its time.

This is the consequence of the depressive's way of looking at the world, and by conceiving of the future as something past, the future is attributed a certain determinism. It is not a question of looking into the future, ascertaining that it *cannot* be any other way, that it *cannot* be any different to what it already is. Rather, what is established is that it *could not* have been any other way. The imagination is caught in a total collapse (bringing to mind Esther to whom capitalism was as given and as natural as the weather itself): "The idea that things could have been different did not cross my mind, *no more than a mountain range, present before my eyes, could vanish to be replaced by a plain*. Consciousness of a total determinism was without a doubt what differentiated us most clearly from our human predecessors."[69] However, there is further cruelty to the ending: In contrast to the compound past (*passé composé*), which indicates a completed action, the French imperfect (*imparfait*) is a descriptive past tense, which, in its lexical definition, indicates an ongoing state of being or a repeated or incomplete action. In *The Possibility of an Island*, this specific grammatical tense can thus be perceived as highlighting how the emptiness or past-ness of the future is not something over and done with. In its very past-ness the future is precisely not past;[70] the effect is rather one of a spectral presence. The lost future is there: it is a mountain, it is real, or rather, it *was* real. This is what is meant by the ultimate words: *La vie était réelle.* Life was real.

Scene 4. Into the tunnel, out of the tunnel (Submission)

...the day before I left, as I made my usual visit to the Chapel of Our Lady, I happened on a reading of Péguy [...] I was in a strange state. It seemed the Virgin was rising from her pedestal and growing in the air. The baby Jesus seemed ready to detach himself from her, and it seemed to me that all he had to do was raise his right hand and the pagans and idolators would be destroyed, and the keys to the world restored to him, "as its lord, its possessor, and its master" [...] Or maybe I was just hungry. I'd forgotten to eat the day before, and possibly what I should do was go back to my hotel and sit down to a few ducks' legs instead of falling down between the pews in an attack of mystical hypoglycemia. I thought again of Huysmans, of the sufferings and doubts of his conversion, and of his desperate desire to be part of a religion.[71]

The year is 2022, a groundbreaking election is taking place in France, the Muslim Brotherhood come to power, endorsed by the socialists and almost everyone else except the Front National, and their candidate Ben Abbes is elected the new president of the French Republic. However, the protagonist of Michel Houellebecq's novel *Submission* of 2015, François – a depressed 44-year-old, specialist in the decadent Catholic writer Jaris-Karl Huysmans – decides to leave Paris for the time being. The capital is in tumult and his only real love, a Jewish woman named Myriam, has gone to Israel due to the escalation of the situation. François heads for the pilgrimage city of Rocamadour, where he makes a daily habit of visiting the Notre Dame church with its carved wood icon of the Black Madonna. It is here, during one of his daily visits, that François happens upon a reading of Péguy, the French Catholic poet. Sitting in front of the Virgin while the poems are being read and performed, he experiences a gleam of spirituality to the point of witnessing the Black Madonna "rising from her pedestal and growing in the air." One would almost think that this is a religious experience equivalent to that of Huysmans. But as always the situation is punctured by Houellebecq: Perhaps François is just hungry and should just go back to his hotel "and sit down to a few ducks' legs." Spirituality and a low blood sugar level are all much of a muchness. Nevertheless, the scene remains significant; in fact, Houellebecq has called it a key scene in as much as it really brings a persistent – albeit somewhat suspect – Houellebecqian subject to the fore: The issue of religion, spirituality, belief and faith. As Norwegian writer Karl Ove Knausgård accentuates in his review of the novel in *The New York Times,* its central question is: "What does it mean to be a human being without faith?"[72] However, in Houellebecq this question is inseparable from a depressive perspective, position and problem. For example, the way in which a sudden need for religion or spirituality arises and makes itself felt within the precarious, painful state that depression is, even in a person who had no faith to begin with. This is the first question: How can depression be understood as a spiritual crisis, a crisis of faith in the future? The second question is how this crisis manifests itself at a personal and political level simultaneously and how these two levels are interrelated. The third and final question is whether religion or spirituality can really be said to constitute a cure in the world of Houellebecq? Having already shown how technology and science in the novels *Atomised* and *The Possibility of an Island* did not solve anything, I ask if religion and spirituality, in contrast, are able to indicate – as the subtitle on François' dissertation on Huysmans reads – a road *out of the tunnel?*

Huysmans and Houellebecq

But why, after all, does François have any interest in a writer as religious as Huysmans? At one point in *Submission* François states: "I was almost completely lacking in spiritual fibre."[73] A theme elaborated elsewhere as well, where François describes how an atheist reader of the religious and spiritual adventures of Huysmans' protagonist Durtal easily ends up getting bored. Yet the study of Huysmans is what François has dedicated his (academic) life to. On Houellebecq's part as an author, there is a profound preoccupation with, if not respect for, such adventures, not only in *Submission* but in his other works as well. In *The Possibility of an Island,* for instance, the comedian Daniel1, explaining the reason he has never introduced sects such as the Elohimites into one of his sketches, declares: "[I]t is easy to make jokes about human beings [...] but when they give the impression of being animated by deep faith, by something that goes beyond the survival instinct, the mechanism breaks down, and laughter in principle is stopped."[74]

That must be why Houellebecq, in *Submission,* lets François read and write about Huysmans, but also follow in his footsteps. François not only pays a visit to the Chapel of Our Lady in Rocamadour, but later spends time in Ligugé Abbey, to which Huysmans had also withdrawn a century or so before, though this is no success for François either. Both François and all of Huysmans' alter egos feel utterly repelled by that which their respective worlds have to offer them. Toward the end of Huysmans' so-called decadence Bible, *Against Nature* (À rebours (1888)), the main character and nobleman Jean Floressas des Esseintes, he of a "libidinous past" – having expressed his dismay with "the caliphate of the counter, the rule of the Rue du Sentier [...] the ungodly tabernacle of the Bank!" – cries out: "May you crumble into dust, Society; old world, may expire!"[75] Significantly, des Esseintes is not so much hero as anti-hero. On the verge of perishing in his own aestheticism, he tries to retire from the world in order to find some spiritual comfort in the Catholic faith, which is not too easy. "It was obvious," the

53

narrator of *Against Nature* declares, "there remained no haven, no shore where he might shelter."[76] Just like Huysmans himself, des Esseintes is a skeptic – he has a strong distrust of any kind of faith – who wants to believe. On the very last page of the novel, Des Esseintes, in a state of utter desperation and misery, turns "for help and comfort to Schopenhauer's consoling precepts; he repeated to himself the painful axiom of Pascal," and it is then that he realizes that it is no good. "He finally realized that the arguments of pessimism were incapable of giving him comfort, that only the impossible belief in a future life would give him peace."[77] *Against Nature* thus ends with a desperate plea: "Lord, take pity on the Christian who doubts, on the unbeliever who longs to believe, on the galley-slave of life who is setting sail alone, at night, under a sky no longer lit, now, by the consoling beacons of the ancient hope!"[78] This plea became the point of departure of Huysmans' ensuing works – *Lá-bas* (1891), *En route* (1895), *La Cathédrale* (1898) and *L'Oblat* (1903) – all of which feature and follow the character Durtal, his spiritual journey and conversion to Catholicism. This is indeed the way out of the tunnel, no longer lit "by the consoling beacons of the ancient hope."

Overall, des Esseintes is described as a sick spirit, a man whose illness is – in keeping with the times – construed as a nervous exhaustion: In other words, a somewhat typical case of fin-de-siècle neurasthenia. Huysman was deeply engrossed in the new psychiatric concepts and diagnoses of the time as put forth by scientists such as Alexandre Axenfelt and Eugéne Bouchut, and convinced that the remedy to these illnesses was of a religious or spiritual nature, specifically the Catholic faith. In this context, the fundamental point is that an intimate relation between despair and belief, between pathology and religion or spirituality, is at work in the work of Huysmans.[79] This is the case in Houellebecq too. But whereas Huysmans' novel *Against Nature* features the pathology of neurasthenia, Houellebecq stages the pathology of depression.

The suicide of Europe

There is a long and great tradition of studying the relation between depression and religion, even if, as Stanley W. Jackson shows in *Melancholia and Depression: From Hippocratic Times to Modern Times*, religious melancholy lost its validity as a clinical category around 1900. Robert Burton devoted the final chapter of his monumental *The Anatomy of Melancholy* (1621) to the subject. Though he was mainly concerned with instances of enthusiastic, superstitious, delirious religiosity, he did reflect at some length on what he called *religious melancholy in defect:* "that other extreme, or defect of this love of God," an entirely "monstrous" or "poisoned" melancholy.[80] For Burton, religious despair is simply the most terrible sickness; "it is more than melancholy in the highest degree."[81]

What is even more interesting and relevant is that William James and Karl Jaspers – two more or less contemporaries of Huysmans – were preoccupied with the rise of secularism (or what in France is called laïcité) and the relation between depression and spiritual despair within that emerging historical formation. For Jaspers, in his *General Psychopathology*, spiritual despair and loss of faith inhere in the experience of depression. In James' *Varieties of Religious Experience* (1902), there is a chapter named "The Sick Souls," in which at one point he describes, translates and quotes a French example of religious melancholy, reportedly an autobiographical experience from 1872 that James disguised as that of a French correspondent.[82] The account begins:

> While in this state of philosophic pessimism and general depression of spirits about my prospects, I went out one evening into a dressing-room in the twilight to procure some article that was there; when suddenly there fell upon me

without any warning, just as if it came out of the darkness, a horrible fear of my own existence.[83]

And it ends with the words: "I have always thought that this experience of melancholia of mine had a religious bearing."[84] This is why James talks about *the sick soul,* summarizing the whole problematic in his usual emphatic and elegant manner: "Here is the real core of the religious problem: Help! Help!"[85]

Neither James nor Jaspers were particularly interested in the spiritual crisis of depression as a purely individual phenomenon. They both developed their respective analysis as a critical diagnosis of the society at that time. As such the pathological problem they anatomized must be understood as a symptom of the *Zeitgeist,* of an age "poor in faith" as Jaspers puts it. And just as the neurasthenia of des Esseintes in *Against Nature* is of course also a neuro-pathological symptom of the society of his day,[86] the personal spiritual crisis that is part of François' depression is brought to address a more general and historical spiritual crisis in *Submission.* "Without Christianity, the European nations had become bodies without souls – zombies," the character Rediger explains to François at one point, before adding: "Europe had already committed suicide."[87] An idea expressed repeatedly in the book is that atheism is doomed. Though Houellebecq is well known for his ridicule of spiritual movements such as the Elohimites in *The Possibility of an Island* – in the conversational book with Bernard-Henri Lévy, *Public Enemies,* he talks derogatorily about "ecological fundamentalism," "left-wing alter-globalization" and "half-witted New Age cults"[88] – these movements only testify to the fact that the Western world faces a fundamental problem according to Houellebecq: The problem of religion. In an interview with Sylvian Bourmeau made in connection with the publication of *Submission* and published in *The Paris Review,* Houellebecq stated: "I think there is a real need for God and that the return of religion is not a slogan, but a reality, and that it is very much on the rise." In *Submission*, this is what the Muslim Brotherhood's presidential candidate Ben Abbes has understood better than anyone among the political elite: "Ben Abbes had kept his distance from the anti-capitalist left. He understood that the pro-growth right had won the 'war of ideas,' that young people today had become *entrepreneurs*, and that no one saw any alternative to the free market."[89] Thus, Ben Abbes is the only one who sizes up the contemporary crisis of faith, offering people something to believe in; something, indeed, to submit themselves to. It is in this sense that Islam or the so-called and apparently imminent Islamization of France is, as Knausgård notes in his review, "merely a consequence." However, the problem with Knausgård's otherwise perceptive review is not only that he fails to note the relation between depression and religion; he also subscribes to a fairly conventional and conservative analysis of the novel, or at least subscribes to what could be perceived as the novel's own conservative diagnosis of the contemporary situation: "This is what the novel is about, an entire culture's enormous loss of meaning, its lack of, or highly depleted, faith, a culture in which the ties of community are dissolving."[90] Knausgård thus reduces the spiritual question at work in *Submission* to a question of culture; to an existential loss of meaning or a cultural loss of values. What Knausgård fails to consider, in other words, is the role of the political economy, which is to say, the capitalist libidinal economy and the ways in which it both depends upon and profroundly alters our very innermost being, our beliefs, affects and desires, our brain, our spirit, our soul.[91] The personal crisis of François is symptomatic of a broader, political and spiritual crisis in the Western world. His depression is a pathology which in the eyes of the novel has favorable conditions under the current neoliberal organization of a society that has both become totally secularized and seems to have arrived at the end of history: It is impossible to believe in or imagine anything other than what already is. Within this kind of spiritual misery, all that remains in which to invest energy is the given, pre-established competitive field.[92]

A shelter for bodies without souls?

There is another obvious but nonetheless important difference between Huysmans' des Esseintes and Houellebecq's François: Whereas the former is an aristocrat, the latter is a more ordinary man, despite being an academic. However, the most crucial difference between des Esseintes and perhaps especially Durtal *and* François is that François evidently never arrives at the point at which it becomes possible to believe. In the aforementioned – rather unbearable – book by Houellebecq and Lévy, the conversation eventually turns toward Victor Hugo, whom reportedly once suffered a terrible period of depression. Here Houellebecq ponders the question: "[W]hat if it was spiritualism that brought him through it?"[93] The same question seems to guide *Submission,* even if nothing more comes of it than a skewed attempt to get out of the depressive condition – to get out of the tunnel so to speak – by way of religion and spirituality. The realization that spirituality and religion are necessary is certainly present, but the necessity does not carry a possibility within it, at least not on an individual level. It remains unavailable to François, as the scene in the Chapel of Our Lady in Rocamadour shows. At a collective, societal level the religious solution leads, at best, to an Islamic state with polygamy and a religious education system. This is not a pure and unequivocal dystopia. In the interview mentioned above Houellebecq even "admitted" that "France is not committing suicide at all. What's more, for people to convert is a sign of hope, not a threat. It means they aspire to a new kind of society."

That this issue is not decidable is not a cliché but a concrete consequence of the temporal perspective and the grammatical tense that increasingly mark the final part of the novel, where the tense changes from past to future conditional tense (*le conditionelle*), designating a situation's occurrence as uncertain or conditioned. "A few more weeks would go by," the last chapter thus begins and continues in this tense for the few remaining pages of the novel, which ends with a slightly modulated version of Edith Piaf's famous line "Je ne regrette rien": "Rather like my father a few years before, I'd be given another chance; and it would be the chance at a second life, with very little connection to the old one. I would have nothing to mourn."[94] For the first time in Houellebec's *oeuvre*, the time and point of narration does not transcend or overhaul the end of the action, which creates a final ambiguity different from his other books. There is no saying what is actually going to happen and how this is to be viewed and judged. But what remains unambiguously clear is that François, whether in the Chapel of Our Lady or elsewhere, is incapable of undertaking the absurd leap of faith required of him. Rather, he trudges along into a more or less unknown future. And though there is no discernible difference between a critical blood sugar level and a spiritual experience, this is perhaps less to be read as a satirical rejection of the depressive problematic – the depressed person's crisis of faith – than as a cementation of the problem. Rather than emphasizing the problem's *irrelevance*, the scene may be interpreted as highlighting its *importance* and *insistence*. For there is only one thing more disheartening than bodies without souls who seek shelter in an act of spiritual submission: Depressed people who are unable – or unwilling? – to find shelter anywhere at all.

A reviewer wrote of *Against Nature* that "[a]fter such a book, the only thing left for the author is to choose between the muzzle of a pistol and the foot of the cross. The choice is made." In *Submission* that choice has not yet been made: François is still standing there, between the muzzle of a pistol and the foot of the cross.

Old age and the art of depression (Threshold)

In the works of Houellebecq, depression crystallizes as a time in itself, or rather an age in itself. The problem that is present(ed) in all of his books is that of old age. The world in Houellebecq is an old and weary world and, accordingly, all of his characters are always already too old, even in *Whatever* where the protagonist is only 30. *The Possibility of an Island*, for instance, is a novel concerned with "the unbearable nature of the mental suffering caused by old age."[95] As mentioned, between the divorce with his first and only wife and his entrance into the sect of the Elohimites, Daniel1 has a brief relationship with the very young and attractive Esther, which of course does not last long. In a particularly devastating scene, Esther is throwing a party for all her young friends, with copious amounts of cocaine, and the depressed Daniel is feeling helplessly old; Esther as good as disowns him and at the end of the party, nearing dawn, Daniel finds himself outside next to a swimming pool, masturbating: "I was evidently on the home stretch."[96]

This depressing experience is inextricably linked to the contemporary consumer capitalism, that, according to the narrator of *The Possibility of an Island*, is "turning youth into the supremely desirable commodity." As the French collective of artists and activists Tiqqun suggest in their book *Preliminary Materials for a Theory of the Young-Girl*, the young girl is the ultimate model or figure for capitalism today. Consumers are also producers, they invest in themselves, realize themselves, and no one more perfectly than the young girl. In this game, which makes up a generalized state of competition, old men are the emphatic losers. In the end, being old and being depressed amounts to the same thing, unless you are both old *and* depressed; then you are really on the home stretch. It is, indeed, no country for old men.

Alain Ehrenberg has drawn attention to the fact that the depressive is in a sense always prematurely old, but it is Franco "Bifo" Berardi whose reflections provide the possibility for getting to the bottom of this. In several works, Berardi has tried to arrive at an understanding of depression that takes as its point of departure the work of Deleuze and, in particular, Guattari. As Berardi himself points out, there is something paradoxical about this endeavor, since the framework of Deleuze and Guattari leaves almost no room for a consideration of depression, yet what Berardi tries to show is that Deleuze and Guattari did in fact deal with depression at one particular place in their joint work, albeit somewhat unknowingly or implicitly. The place Berardi has in mind is the beginning of the concluding chapter of Deleuze and Guattari's last joined work, *What is Philosophy*: "Old age is this very weariness: then, there is either a fall into mental chaos outside of the plane of composition or a falling-back on ready-made opinions, on clichés that reveal that an artist, no longer able to create new sensations, no longer knowing how to preserve, contemplate, and contract, no longer has anything to say."[97]

Berardi re-frames and re-contextualizes this description of old age as a description of depression, which I fully agree with. But whereas Berardi mentions Jonathan Franzen's novel *The Corrections* as a paradigmatic example of the old age of depression, I want to point to Houellebecq (whom Berardi actually writes about in his latest book, *Futurability: The Age of Impotence and the Horizon of Possibility*). The essential difference is this one: The collapse or disinvestment of desire is the problem of depression, but the solution to this problem is not an abandonment of desire; rather, it is its reinvestment, a new trajectory of desire, or – in the Deleuzian/Guattarian vocabulary – a deterritorialization of desire. Desire is the pharmakon: Poison and cure. The problem according to Berardi, then, is not desire per se, as it is in Houellebecq: In his novels, desire is not something to be deterritorialized but something to be discarded. In the universe of Houellebecq, *everything begins with the end of desire.*

Significantly, the remarks made by Deleuze and Guattari on old age relate specifically to one of the pillars of *What is Philosophy*; namely art. The question they raise is: What does the artist do with old age? How does he or she handle it? Here Berardi, usually a pure pessimist, is quite optimistic on behalf of art. He often ends up emphasizing art's potential to compose the chaos of old age, to show a way out of the labyrinth, to offer new ways for the imagination to go. In *The Uprising* he argues that poetry in particular has the capacity to function as a source of salvation. But what if depressive literature does not function as the opening of an imaginary field, but rather as evidence of the immediate and total collapse of the very faculty of imagination? What if the goal of the writing and language in question is not to reinvest desire but to remove it? What if literature as a potential remedy is not only part of the disease but one of its symptoms? What are we left with then? The answer seems simple: Michel Houellebecq and his depressive and radically symptomatological literature. Indeed, his novels seem to sink into the old age of depression; they appear to accept – or cannot but accept – "a falling-back on ready-made opinions, on clichés that reveal that an artist, no longer able to create new sensations, no longer knowing how to preserve, contemplate, and contract, no longer has anything to say." Here, the question is not so much how art presents the problem of depression but how depression presents a problem for art.

This question pertains to the distance or lack of distance in Houellebecq's body of work, i.e. the position and point of view of narration. The scholarship on Houellebecq often emphasizes the distanced voice of the narrators, or the ways in which they – allegedly – observe society from the outside. Thus, in a recent book, *Michel Houellebecq: Humanity and its aftermath*, the author states that "[t]he point of view appears, on numerous occasions, almost anthropological, or ethnological – our society is observed *as though from the outside* precisely because Houellebecq's narrators do not feel themselves to be fully a part of it."[98] However, my point is exactly the opposite: The distance to which all the works of Houellebecq evidently testify is *not* a distance from without but a distance from *within*: a distance created and constituted by depressive collapse, and no less great than a distance from the outside. To repeat the cogent lines from Andrew Solomon's *Noonday Demon*: "We are depressed not because we are so far removed from what we want, but because we are merged with it."

This of course has consequences for what form of resistance it is possible – and meaningful – to envisage. This is why it is difficult, especially for left-leaning critics, to read Houellebecq. Due to the lack of distance from without, the lack of autonomy, and the lack of an outside, one is easily led to believe that he is a reactionary (he himself wrote in *Atomised* that all great writers are reactionaries). There is no asymmetrical perspective with regards to the object observed and written about, only a total and absolutely symmetrical symptomatology, which means that the responses expressed in his books – as reactions to the problems articulated within them – must also be read as symptoms themselves. Even Houellebecq's utopian scenes are thus evidence of a depressive imagination and the utopian models proposed – technology, religion etc. – are not *solutions* to depression, but *symptoms* of depression.

Before leaving the subject for good, one might make a Jamesonian objection. In *In Archaeologies of the Future: The Desire Called Utopia and Other Science Fictions,* Fredric Jameson writes that science fiction is not at all about the capacity to "keep the future alive, even in imagination. On the contrary, its deepest vocation is over and over again to demonstrate and to dramatize our incapacity to imagine the future."[99] In that sense, Houellebecq's work could be viewed as the perfect example of a truly utopian work – because his books seem to demonstrate Jameson's conception of utopia as "a necessary failure of imagination" and this failure as a kind of reversed Pyrrhic victory – reminiscent of Beckett: "Ever tried. Ever failed. No matter. Try Again. Fail again. Fail better." But Houellebecq goes in the opposite and more literal direction: For him a failure is a failure is a failure. There is no utopian imperative or impulse left. All that remains is a depressed and depressing work of fiction that bears witness to the collapsed space of an impotent imagination: The future has contracted to a zero point, and this is precisely where everything in the fiction of Houellebecq begins and ends. However, the counter to the potential Jamesonian objection might be even more radically formulated: For Houellebecq it does not really make sense to engage in the discussion – dystopian or utopian, failure or success? – using a human scale. This is what such discussions, quite understandably, tend to be characterized by: Is this or that future a good or bad thing *for us*, as human beings? But this is precisely not the central question in Houellebecq, insofar as the very point from which such an evaluation could be conducted is dislocated and displaced beyond any human point of view. Strictly speaking the ending of *The Possibility of an Island* is not aimed or addressed at us, the contemporary human readers, or if it is, its purpose is only to underline our inevitable and essential irrelevance for the future.[100] The reader of Houellebecq is confronted solely by dry ascertainment, a matter-of-fact extrapolation of contemporary conditions, and the depressive recognition that life ends and the human as we know it will disappear. That the future of humanity is a future without humanity. As J. G. Ballard once asked in his manifesto "Notes from Nowhere": "Does the angle between two walls have a happy ending?"

What seems certain is that art is no more able to offer a way out of – or a therapeutic cure for – depression than technology and science or religion and spirituality. Indeed, this should not be in the least surprising given that the protagonist of *Platform* had already declared that his conclusion is "that art cannot change lives. At least not mine."[101] Perhaps art is not able to change life. Perhaps art is actually complicit in the contemporary misery in a variety of ways – and the novels of Houellebecq certainly are that, not least due to the method of symptomatology and the imitation from the inside, whereby, for example, a tired world equals a tired syntax. However, Houellebecq's novels avoid partaking in what Lovecraft calls bland or smirk optimism. That much is clear. The depressive position and perspective prompt Houellebecq to make life – again in the words of Lovecraft – a "thousandfold more hideous," a thousandfold more depressing than it already is. The goal is not relief or reparation, but intensification and multiplication. The only medicine he offers is the assurance that there is no medicine.[102]

Chapter 2

And then nothing turned itself inside out – David Foster Wallace

Introduction

In some oft-quoted lines from his famous 1993 interview with Larry McCaffery, David Foster Wallace declared:

> Look man, we'd probably most of us agree that these are dark times, and stupid ones, but do we need fiction that does nothing but dramatize how dark and stupid everything is? In dark times, the definition of good art would seem to be art that locates and applies CPR to those elements of what's human and magical that still live and glow despite the times' darkness.[1]

The writer from whom Wallace is explicitly distancing himself in this passage is Bret Easton Ellis who, according to Wallace, has chosen the easy – and in every respect cynical – solution: "If readers simply believe the world is stupid and shallow and mean, then Ellis can write a mean shallow stupid novel that becomes a mordant deadpan commentary on the badness of everything."[2] Wallace might as well have been talking about Michel Houellebecq. In clear contrast to Houellebecq, who seems to be content with merely giving an account of the depressive experience as a way of unveiling the world as it is – thereby letting his literature be almost absolutely symmetrical with and symptomatic of this very world – Wallace is convinced that literature has to be an "illumination," a cure, a therapy, a kind of CPR as it were; the critical diagnosis is not enough in itself.

This is the general framework for the following chapter on David Foster Wallace. Scene one and scene two focus rather exclusively on the experience of depression as it is made manifest and expressed in the short story "The Depressed Person" from *Brief Interviews with Hideous Men* (1999) and *Infinite Jest* (1996) respectively, through the nameless protagonist of the former and the character of Kate Gompert in the latter. It is not surprising that depression was a major concern of Wallace's literary work – from his first published story "The Planet Trillaphon As It Stands In Relation To the Bad Thing" which appeared in the college journal *Amherst Review* in 1984 to *The Pale King*, published posthumously in 2011 – given that Wallace suffered from episodes of deep depression for most of his adult life, which ended when he killed himself in 2008. However, my concerns in this chapter are strictly textual, and what follows from the analysis of the two scenes is that depression in Wallace is characterized by a loss of empathy, by a loss of the other. There is temporal aspect to this loss, insofar as the other, as Emmanuel Levinas makes clear, is a category of futurity: "[t]he other is the future. The very relation to the other is the relation to the future."[3]

For Wallace, however, the problem of depression and empathy is related to a problem of *addiction*. All of the characters in *Infinite Jest* are addicts in one way or another, and a central part of the novel takes places at the Ennet House Drug and Alcohol Recovery House, wittily footnoted "Redundancy sic." The relation between depression and addiction is of course well established within psychiatric research: Substance abuse is common among depressive patients, and depressive incidents are, in turn, frequently reported among substance abusers, which is why depression and addiction are sometimes referred to as a double demon. However, what is singular to his works is the way in which they rotate around an axis of self and other, subject and object, and exhibit a sort of cruel double bind. On the one hand, if the relation to the other or the object becomes too strong, the risk is an addictive relation, total immersion (a favored word by Wallace), a hedonistic pursuit of pleasure, or a never-ending quest for recognition from others, whom, for their part, also hope desperately to be perceived and recognized by other others, who in turn seek recognition and so on, in "an endless funhouse hall of mirrors" (to quote from the posthumous novel *The Pale King*). On the other hand, if the relation to the other or the object becomes too weak, the risk is depression, anhedonia, total withdrawal, an enclosed and enfolded self, a world with no mirrors at all. Pick your poison. This is the subject of scene three.

What is the cure, if indeed there is one? That is the question that guides the fourth and final scene. Whereas the response in Houellebecq was ontological, concerning the very being of human beings – or alternatively, a post-human form of being – the response in Wallace has a more ethico-spiritual character, pertaining to the being of the other. It raises issues of love, belief and infinity. Thus, in this fourth scene I turn to "B.I. #20 12-96. New Haven CT," the brutal, yet somehow rather beautiful, penultimate story in *Brief Interviews with Hideous Men*. It is a story about empathy, but the empathy evinced in the story goes beyond any conventional understanding. Though some readers of Wallace – and even Wallace himself – at times seem satisfied with viewing empathy, quite trivially, as the affective and imaginative operation of putting oneself in the proverbial other's shoes, I show how it is much more complicated than that. To this end, I draw Kierkegaard and his highly original reading of the parable of the Good Samaritan in *Works of Love*, so that this particular story by Wallace can be read as a story about presupposing the capacity for love and empathy *in* the other rather than about practicing a love *of* or an empathy *for* the other. Even or especially in cases where the other, the neighbor, is not necessarily a nice guy or a lovable creature, but more often than not a monster, an alien, an unlovable and hideous man.

Scene 1. Zero sense of empathy ("The Depressed Person")

The depressed person was in terrible and unceasing emotional pain and the impossibility of sharing or articulating this pain was itself a component of the pain and a contributing factor in its essential horror [...]

The friends whom the depressed person reached out to for support and tried to open up to and share at least the contextual shape of her unceasing psychic agony and feelings of isolation with numbered around half a dozen and underwent a certain amount of rotation. The depressed person's therapist – who had earned both a terminal graduate degree and a medical degree, and who was the self-professed exponent of a school of therapy which stressed the cultivation and regular use of a supportive peer-community in any endogenously depressed adult's journey toward healing – referred to these female friends as the depressed person's Support System. The approximately half-dozen rotating members of this Support System tended to be either former acquaintances from the depressed person's childhood or else girls she had roomed with at various stages of her school career, nurturing and comparatively undamaged women who now lived in all manner of different cities and whom the depressed person often had not seen in person for years and years, and whom she often called late in the evening, long-distance, for sharing and support and just a few well-chosen words to help get her some realistic perspective on the day's despair and get centered and gather together the strength to fight through the emotional agony of the next day, and to whom, when she telephoned, the depressed person always began by saying that she apologized if she was dragging them down or coming off as boring or self-pitying or repellent or taken them away from their, active, vibrant, largely pain-free long-distance lives.[4]

Within these endless and interlaced spirals, the depressed person of David Foster Wallace's "The Depressed Person," from the short story collection *Brief Interviews with Hideous Men* from 1999, appears before the reader in all her emotional agony and spiritual despair. Unbearably self-conscious and narcissistically self-centered, she is unable to communicate the pain of her depression. The female protagonist has indeed lost any sense of the other. Yet "The Depressed Person" is in fact an atypical text from Wallace's hand in that it does not seek to offer any cure or CPR; it provides no resynchronized rhythm, nor recovery of the other.

The depressed person's obsessive refrain

The story is essentially a loop. There is neither a beginning nor end to the story, nor to the woman's depression. It goes on and on, though she tries everything she can to get help and get out of it. She is on a vast range of medications: Paxil, Zoloft, Prozac, Tofranil, Welbutrin, Elavil. She has a therapist. She reaches out to her friends, to her so-called support system. In this story, then, Wallace shows his intimate familiarity with the language of cognitive therapy, endogenous depression, etiological models and emergent psychopharmacology. He also shows that nothing really works: the depressed person calls her friends but is painfully aware of "what a joyless burden" she must be, as she cannot help but point out, and she makes sure to say to her friends that they absolutely must tell her "the very *second*" they were "getting bored or frustrated or repelled" or decided they "had other more urgent or interesting things to do."[5] However, she is also very well aware of "how pathetic such a need for reassurance might come off to someone, how it could all too possibly be heard not as an open invitation to get off the telephone but actually as a needy, self-pitying, contemptibly manipulative plea for the friend *not* to get off the telephone, *never* to get off the telephone."[6] It does not take the reader long to realize that the depressed person not only draws on her friends, but exploits their empathy and emotional support, an exploitation that is not mitigated but maximized by her self-conscious effort to be open about it. From her helpless and powerless position, she attempts to control the situation and leaves little or no breathing space for her listeners – nor for the readers of the story.

At the same time, the depressed person is so thoroughly self-centered in her pain that she has no understanding nor empathy for anyone other than herself. When her therapist dies, she thinks only about how that affects her therapeutic process, and how inconvenient it is from her perspective. She is utterly unable to "feel or identify any real feelings within herself for the therapist."[7] Earlier, she confesses to her support system that, although they have spent hours and hours talking to each other, she has not once "asked for the therapist's loved ones' names."[8] As for her support system, one of them, "a surpassingly generous and nurturing mother of two in Bloomfield Hills, Michigan," is actually terminally ill and undergoing chemotherapy for "a virulent blastoma," but the depressed person does not care.[9] Or rather, she does not know (which is of course even worse), as she has been too preoccupied with herself to even consider the simple question of how the others in her network are doing. It stands to reason, though, that even if she had known about her friend's terrible condition, she would probably not have felt anything in this case either, except perhaps a slight annoyance. What the depressed person values about this particular terminally ill friend is that she is "not only almost always at home but also enjoyed nearly unlimited conflict-free availability and time to share on the telephone, for which the depressed person was always careful to enter a daily prayer of gratitude in her Feelings

Journal."[10] Later the depressed person does admit to this friend that she is "frightened for herself, for as it were '[her] *self* – i.e. for her own so-called 'character' or 'spirit' or as it were 'soul', i.e. for her own capacity for basic human empathy and compassion and caring," before continuing with the question: "What kind of person could seem to feel nothing – '*Nothing*', she emphasized – for anyone but herself? Maybe not *ever*?"[11] A person feeling nothing for others is, as Marshall Boswell observes, a nothing, a void.[12]

Reading "The Depressed Person" is an absolutely claustrophobic experience. At no time is it possible to step outside the stream of self-consciousness with its recursive sentences and dizzying syntax, the effect of which has been well described by Zadie Smith: "To read those spiral sentences is to experience that dread of circularity embedded in the old joke about recursion (*to understand recursion you must first understand recursion*), as well as the existential vertigo we feel when we stand before two mirrors."[13] In her otherwise perceptive reading, however, Smith does not mention how the story's formal features could and should be seen as symptoms of the depression at work in the story. The speech of the depressed person as a character and the style of "The Depressed Person" as a story betray a thoroughly depressed rhythm, testifying to what Franco "Bifo" Berardi terms the *obsessive refrain* of the psychopathology of depression.[14]

Within the psychiatric literature, in particular phenomenological psychiatry, it is not uncommon to describe mental illnesses in terms of a rhythmic disturbance or dissonance: Thomas Fuchs, for one, speaks of the desynchronized rhythm of depression, meaning a depressive rhythm that is out of synch with the rhythm of the surrounding world. Accordingly, to Fuchs the purpose of the therapeutic process is to resynchronize being, which is to say, "to re-establish [the depressed patient's] protensivity" and "to give rhythm to everyday life."[15] Philosophically, the concept of rhythm stems from Henri Lefebvre's *Rhythmanalysis*, wherein rhythm plays a central role in the analysis of everyday life: "Everywhere where there is interaction between a place, a time and expenditure of energy, there is rhythm."[16] Rhythms are thus at work in all parts of life, but sometimes the basic rhythm is interrupted or disturbed, thereby creating a pathological form of rhythm that Lefebvre dubs *arrhythmia* ("arythmie" in French). Rhythm is of course also a musical term, apotheosized in pop music as the *refrain*. Inspired by Lefebvre and even more by Félix Guattari, Franco "Bifo" Berardi has ventured into an exploration of the relation between rhythm/refrain and psychopathologies such as depression. "The refrain," he writes,

> is above all a musical phrase that returns in the course of a song: a phrase that, in returning, constructs and brings forth the complex rhythm. It is a factor of assemblage: by constructing rhythm and bringing forth the song's complex rhythm, the refrain functions as the structuring element in language, in existential behavior, and in history.[17]

The refrain is thus more than a designation of a musical phenomenon; according to Berardi it pertains to the very rhythmic relation between *Organismus* and *Umwelt*. The refrain is what holds together a world or a life; it sustains relations to other people and to one's self. What happens in the depressive state is that this rhythm hardens and becomes compulsive, as when you have a particular piece of music on the brain: It sticks in your head, in your body and you cannot get it out. On and on it goes, round and round.

This is literally how "The Depressed Person" operates as a text: It consists of a series of suffocating repetitions, in which the narrator merely mimes the thoughts and speech acts of the depressed protagonist. Formally and stylistically "The Depressed Person" bears the stamp of the compulsive and obsessive refrain of depression from which there is no escape.

"Our own tiny skull-sized kingdoms"

In his *General Psychopathology* (1946), Karl Jaspers calls attention to the *pathological and clinical* problem of "a failure of empathy."[18] Moreover, he regards the problem of empathy as an integral part of the therapeutic practice, insofar as there can be no direct access to the psychic experiences of others, which implies that there must be "an act of empathy" on the part of the clinician or psychiatrist in order for him or her to help.[19] Empathy is thus simultaneously a diagnostic and a therapeutic category, an epistemological and an ethical problem.[20] For Wallace it is, however, a *contemporary and cultural* problem as well. After all, all of *Brief Interviews with Hideous Men* are explorations of people –mostly men – who have zero sense of empathy. There is a man who leaves his girlfriend because she has been too explicit about her fear that he might leave her, which thus becomes a self-fulfilling prophesy and a very neat excuse for the man in question; there is another man who takes advantage of a girl when she is not picked up at the airport by the love of her life; and there is a man who uses his crippled arm as an "asset" to get more "pussy than a toilet seat."[21] In short, it is a book about people who cannot love or empathize and who, as the book itself formulates it, have severe problems with "other-directedness"[22] – of which the depressed person is the radicalized and pathological instance.

In "The Science of Evil" Simon Baron-Cohen argues that empathy has eroded in our time, the primary consequence of which is "people turning people into objects." "In such a state," he notes, "we relate only to things, or to people as if they were just things."[23] In *Brief Interviews with Hideous Men* this erosion of empathy seems to be the very condition of the violence, sexual abuse and misogyny permeating every fiber of the book. What is lost is precisely the other, or, put another way, what is depicted is how the other is turned into an object, which amounts to one and the same thing. Is the loss of the other or the transformation of the other into an object a consequence of a culture of narcissism? According to several critics, what Wallace tries to capture is a specifically American problem of generalized narcissism.[24] Examples of narcissistic behavior in Wallace are legion, and not only in *Brief Interviews with Hideous Men*. In *Infinite Jest* the whole Incandenza family, the focal point of the novel, is haunted by it. One of the sons, Orin, is sexually aroused by watching himself play American football on TV and the mother, Avril, has to be at the exact center of every room that she finds herself in.[25] In his by now famous commencement speech "This Is Water," which he delivered at Kenyon College in May 2005, Wallace seemed to pick on precisely this image in a passage that discussed "the worship of self": "Our own present culture has harnessed these forces in ways that have yielded extraordinary wealth and comfort and personal freedom. The freedom to be lords of our own tiny skull-sized kingdoms, alone at the center of all creation."[26]

Vicious infinite regress (what is funny and not so funny about "The Depressed Person")

Narcissism and loss of empathy – two crucial factors in depression. What Wallace seems absorbed by in "The Depressed Person" is anatomizing – and ridiculing – the workings of the depressed person's mind, or what some have called the nightmare of consciousness. The consciousness of the consciousness, and the consciousness of the consciousness of the consciousness...The story is an introspection on the depressive process's introspective character. That said, for Wallace, abstract thinking and existential feeling, rationality and affect, and mind and body are two sides of the same coin. The distinction between "I think" and "I feel" is immediately and irreversibly undermined. Any feeling is not only concerned with itself, but also inextricably bound up with the (self)consciousness of this feeling. The (self)consciousness of a feeling thus produces a "new" or intensified feeling. This is the case with the character Cusk from *The Pale King;* a man who sweats an awful lot, which makes him very self-conscious, and in turn makes him sweat even more, making him even more self-conscious and so on and so forth. He fears the sweating, but he also fears the fear, and the fear of the fear, resulting in "an endless funhouse hall of mirrors of fear."[27]

This phenomenon is paradigmatic of what Wallace calls *vicious infinite regress.* The concept features in several of Wallace's stories, such as "Good old neon" from *Oblivion* of 2004, but it is developed more theoretically in *Everything and More,* his book on the mathematical concept of infinity, where Wallace provides the following example of vicious infinite regress:

> You're standing at a corner and the light changes and you try to cross the street. Note the operative "try to." Because before you can get all the way across the street, you obviously have to get halfway across. And before you can get halfway across, you have to get halfway to that halfway point. This is just common sense [...] the sequence has no finite end. Goes on forever. This is the dreaded *regressus in infinitum,* a.k.a. the Vicious Infinite Regress or VIR. What makes it vicious here is that you're required to complete an infinite number of actions before attaining your goal, which – since the whole point of "infinite" is that there is no end to the number of these actions – renders the goal logically impossible. Meaning you can't cross the street.[28]

As with everything else, Wallace's interest in this concept was not purely mathematical; he was particularly preoccupied with the existential implications. Much of his interest in Wittgenstein followed the same pattern. The fundamental question for Wallace became: What would it be like to *live* in the Wittgensteinian world of the *Tractatus*? An inability to cross the street thus translates into an inability to access the help that is needed. One cannot get out of depression. This is the depressed person's painful problem and is one of (self)consciousness, reflection and thinking in general. In *Infinite Jest* it is called "Analysis-Paralysis," or as a slogan of the AA goes in the novel: "My Best Thinking Got Me Here." Consciousness of a given problem is often part of that very problem. Knowledge does not lead to action; the diagnosis does not entail the cure.

Specifically, for the female protagonist of "The Depressed Person," the reader witnesses a gradual intensification and infinitization of her depressed condition in line with the cruel logic indicated above: The more she reaches out to her friends, the more she becomes self-conscious, ashamed and disgusted with herself, prompting her to reach out to her friends even more, making her even more self-conscious, ashamed and disgusted with herself, and so on *ad nauseam, ad absurdum, ad infinitum.* This kind of vicious infinite regress is not only tragic; it is inherently comical.[29] Why? To answer that question, an excursion involving Wallace's relationship to Wittgenstein is necessary.

From beginning to end, Wallace was in a sense a student of Wittgenstein, always trying to live up to the latter's dictum in *Philosophical Investigations*: "The philosopher treats a question; like an illness" – though naturally for Wallace this was transformed into a question of aesthetic or literary methodology. In the same book Wittgenstein wrote: "There is not a single philosophical method, though there are indeed methods, different therapies, as it were." The project of philosophy is thus, simply, "[t] o show the fly the way out of the fly-bottle."[30] Wallace adopts almost completely this ambitious project and original imagery. As already stated, he does not believe that literature should be satisfied with showing how dark the world is; it has to include a therapy or remedy – to apply CPR – which is to say: Show the fly a way out of the bottle, or show the human a way out of the labyrinth. The only issue is that in Wallace's writing, the way *out* of the labyrinth may finally lead deeper and further *into* it;

the abandonment of the self may finally be an affirmation of the self. When Wallace tries to gesture toward an exit – or a way out of the bottle, in Wittgensteinian imagery – there is always the possibility that that exit is in fact the entrance to another bottle. A paradoxical and dark variety of comedy emerges here. This is indeed the comedy of "The Depressed Person." As Wallace wrote himself in an essay on Kafka, whose humor was marked by a "harrowing spirituality" that is deeply relevant here:

> To envision us readers coming up and pounding on this door, pounding and pounding, not just wanting admission but needing it, we don't know what it is but we can feel it, this total desperation to enter, pounding and pushing and kicking, etc. That, finally, the door opens...and it opens outward: we've been inside what we wanted all along. *Das ist komisch.*[31]

What is not *komisch* at all, however, is that the laughter in "The Depressed Person" is directed toward the depressed person herself: The joke is on her alone. According to Berardi, however, the refrains of literature can in themselves constitute a deviation from the hardened, compulsive rhythm of depression. Is that the case in "The Depressed Person"? Does the text succeed where its protagonist fails? These questions are of immense importance, since "The Depressed Person" is not a clinical case but a short story, a work of fiction. As I indicated, I operate under the assumption that Wallace's fiction can be understood in terms of rhythm. By this I mean both the rhythms *in* the text – at the level of content – and the rhythms *of* the text – at the level of form. It is thus not enough to look at how the text *represents* empathy; it is also imperative to consider how and to what extent it *produces* empathy. Here, we are not dealing with the other *in* the text but the other *of* the text, that is, the reader, the implicit "you." This pertains to the literary act of communicating to another person, though often in the form of indirect communication (á la Kierkegaard). To put it bluntly: The goal of Wallace's fiction is to reinvent, rebuild, or repair the relation to the other.

Yet in "The Depressed Person" no such thing occurs; despite all the communicative efforts, there is no "other," no "you." As Judith Butler writes: "If I have lost the conditions of address, if I have no 'you' to address, then I have lost 'myself',"[32] a loss that seems to be what "The Depressed Person" cannot (or will not) overcome. The story produces no empathy. The rhythm in and of the text thus remains desynchronized to the very end, empathy is never restored, the other is not recovered. The depressed person *as a person* risks no empathy (the phrase "no risk of empathy" turns up in *Infinite Jest*[33]) but neither does "The Depressed Person" *as a text* by David Foster Wallace. The depressed protagonist is thoroughly ridiculed, brutally exposed in her depression, narcissism, and unsympathetic behavior and thoughts – often to tremendous comical effect, although the smile stifles at some point. If rhythms, as a character in one of the other stories in the collection *Brief Interviews with Hideous Men* says, are "relations between what you believe and what you believed before,"[34] then "The Depressed Person" remains an utterly a-rhythmic piece of fiction – in spite of its repetitive, obsessive cadence (of course arrhythmia is in itself a kind of rhythm). What this means is that the story reads like a broken record, like a vinyl skipping the whole way through; the story does not pull the emergency brake on the vicious infinite regress. No difference is established, then, between what you believe and what you believed before – and what you believe(d) was and still is: nothing at all.

Scene 2. "It's like horror more than sadness" (Kate Gompert and *Infinite Jest*)

"What I am trying to ask, I think, is whether this feeling you're communicating is the feeling you associate with your depression."

Her gaze moved off. "That's what you guys want to call it, I guess."

The doctor clicked his pen slowly a few times and explained that he's more interested here in what *she* would choose to call the feeling, since it was her feeling.

The resumed study of the movement of her feet. "When people call it that I always get pissed off because I always think *depression* sounds like you just get really sad, you get quiet and melancholy and just like sit quietly by the window sighing or just lying around. A state of not caring about anything. A kind of blue kind of peaceful state." She seemed to the doctor decidedly more animated now, even as she seemed unable to meet his eyes. Her respiration had sped back up. The doctor recalled classic hyperventilatory episodes being characterized by carpopedal spasms, and reminded himself to monitor the patient's hands and feet carefully during the interview for any signs of tetanic contraction, in which case the prescribed therapy would be IV calcium in a saline percentage he would need quickly to look up.

"Well *this*" – she gestured at herself – 'isn't a state. This is a *feeling*. I feel it all over. In my arms and legs."

"That would include your carp – your hands and feet?"

"All *over*. My head, throat, butt. In my stomach. It's all over everywhere. I don't know what I could call it. It's like I can't get enough outside it to call it anything. It's like horror more than sadness. It's more like horror. It's like something horrible is about to happen, the most horrible thing you can imagine – no, worse than you can imagine because there's the feeling that there's something you have to do right away to stop it but you don't know what it is you have to do, and then it's happening, too, the whole horrible time, it's about to happen and also it's happening, all at the same time."[35]

The depressed woman in this story is Kate Gompert from David Foster Wallace's magnum opus of 1996, *Infinite Jest*. With its more than 1000 pages and numerous, endless footnotes the novel is somewhat resistant to a brief summary but: The novel is set in a near future, so altered in terms of political landscape that the US, Canada and Mexico have become The Organization of North American Nations (abbreviated in the novel as ONAN in a not so subtle reference to the biblical figure of Onan) – against which a group of Quebecois wheelchair terrorists stage a sophisticated and violent revolt – and so commercialized that every calendar year is designated by corporate brands – Year of the Whopper, Year of the Perdue Wonderchicken etc. – rather than successive numbers. The main part of the novel takes place in the Year of the Depend Adult Undergarment and has as its central locations the Enfield Tennis Academy (ETA) and Ennet House Drug and Alcohol Recovery House, both situated in Boston, Massachusetts. And 21-year-old Kate Gompert does in fact become a resident at the halfway house, as the drug and alcohol recovery house is colloquially called. However, when we first meet her she is still at a psychiatric clinic on "suicide watch" as a result of her unipolar depression – intimately tied up with her substance abuse of marijuana – and her fourth failed suicide attempt.

The Black Hole of Depression (depression vs. anxiety)

In the scene Kate, curled up on the bed in her room at the clinic, is approached by a doctor who attempts to engage her in conversation about her depressive state. What she is quick to point out in this dialog with the rather uncomprehending doctor, who persistently translates everything she says into his own technocratic language – "The doctor recalled classic hyperventilatory episodes being characterized by carpopedal spasms" – is that for her, depression is a feeling, and not one of sadness but of pain and horror: "It's like horror more than sadness."[36] This horror has something to do with affect (the feeling of sheer physical pain in her "head throat, butt"), with imagination ("the most horrible thing you can imagine") and time ("it's about to happen and also it's happening, all at the same time").

The doctor still does not understand: "So you'd say anxiety is a big part of your depressions," he tries. But no. It is not sadness, nor anxiety.

> "Listen," Kate Gompert said. "Have you ever felt sick? I mean nauseous, like you know you were going to throw up?" The doctor made a gesture like Well sure. "But that's just in your stomach," Kate Gompert said. "It's a horrible feeling but it's just in your stomach […] imagine if you felt that way all over, inside. All through you. Like every cell and every atom or brain-cell or whatever was so nauseous it wanted to throw up, but it couldn't, and you felt that way all the time, and you're sure, you're positive the feeling will never go away, you're going to spend the rest of your natural life feeling like this."[37]

This passage is an almost verbatim copy of Wallace's early and unusually autobiographical story "The Planet Trillaphon as It Stands in Relation to the Bad Thing" from 1984, where depression is, simply, "the Bad Thing." In some emphatic lines the narrator of "The Planet Trillaphon" notes that "it's like having always before you and under you a huge black hole without a bottom, a black, black hole, maybe with vague teeth in it, and then your being part of the hole, so that you fall even when you stay where you are (...maybe when you realize *you're* the hole, nothing else...)."[38] In the same passage – obviously the source of our scene in *Infinite Jest* – he describes the Bad Thing as follows: "Just imagine that, a sickness spread utterly through every bit of you, even the bits of the bits. So that your very...very essence is characterized by nothing other than the feature of sickness; you and the sickness are, as they say, 'one.'"[39] Wallace does not just emphasize the unrepresentable character of depression, but its sheer, all-encompassing and enveloping physical and psychic pain, as well as the fact that depression is not so much a bottomless hole in front or outside of you, as a hole *inside* you; you and the hole are one; you *are* the hole. The thing about depression, according to Wallace, is that it is impossible to get on the outside of it. Depression saturates being; it is a feeling, which takes complete possession of the human being that experiences it. In that sense the allusion to the physical concept of black holes is not out of place, since there is no bottom to a black hole; it simply engulfs you, rips you further and further apart in the dead mass of darkness, where the pull of gravity is so strong that even light cannot escape. It reflects no light.

The feeling of the feeling of depression (depression vs. anhedonia)

This is the reason Kate says that, when she is feeling depressed, she is utterly convinced that the present feeling is going to stretch eternally into the future, and it is impossible to imagine any alternative: "You're positive the feeling will never go away, you're going to spend the rest of your natural life feeling like this." To which the doctor remarks: "And yet this nauseated feeling has come and gone for you in the past, it's passed eventually during prior depressions, Katherine, has it not?" Kate replies: "But when you're in the feeling you forget. The feeling feels like it's always been there and will always be there, and you forget [...] I can't stand feeling like this another second, and the seconds keep coming on and on."[40] The temporal experience Kate expresses here is that her sense of chronology is lost. Past and future blur and time is thus reduced to an entirely frozen time, creating a sense that the feeling of depression is all there is, and always has been and always will be. It is a coming catastrophe that has already taken place and keeps taking place: "It's about to happen and also it's happening." This is the affective and temporal horror of depression in Wallace's work.

At the same time this aspect obviously relates to what was earlier defined as a meta-feeling: a feeling of a feeling. As has already been discussed, depression can be described as the lack of feeling (you do not feel anything) and as a feeling of a feeling (but this feeling of not feeling anything is itself a feeling; indeed, it can feel horrifying not to feel a thing). When she talks about what "the feeling feels like," Kate Gompert seems to be well aware that a given feeling can be felt in various ways and that a lack of feeling can feel terrible. But her problem is not that she does not feel anything. She explicitly states that she would rather "feel nothing than this."

What this translates into, 500 pages later in the novel, is that the kind of clinical depression that Gompert experiences may not quite be understood as anhedonia; an inability "to feel pleasure or attachment to things formerly important," "a kind of emotional novocaine," an anesthetic condition of affective numbness wherein one does not feel a thing.[41] Here, anhedonia is further defined as "a kind of radical abstracting of everything, a hollowing out of stuff that used to have affective content. Terms the undepressed toss around and take for granted as full and fleshy – *happiness, joie de vivre, preference, love* – are stripped to their skeletons and reduced to abstract ideas. They have, as it were, denotation but not connotation." A geometrical transformation or perversion of the immediate *Umwelt* is here brought about to such an extent that "[e]verything becomes an outline of the thing. Objects become schemata. The world becomes a map of the world. An anhedonic can navigate, but has no location. i.e. the anhedonic becomes, in the lingo of Boston AA, Unable To Identify." In short, everything becomes "as moving, all of a sudden, as a theorem of Euclid."[42] This particular understanding of anhedonia, as well as the reference to Euclid, is interesting for at least two reasons. Firstly, the evocation of Euclid in *Infinite Jest* is lifted directly from the passage of William James' *Varieties of Religious Experience* that I mentioned in the chapter on Houellebecq. Here, James quotes a certain Professor Ribot who describes an anhedonic man as being in a state where "[e]very emotion appeared dead within him" and "[t]he thought of his house, of his home, of his wife, and of his absent children moved him as little [...] as a theorem of Euclid."[43] In this state, one simply loses touch with the objects and the others around oneself. Secondly, the passage is undeniably analogous with some symptomatic scenes in the novels of Houellebecq. The scene in *Atomised,* for instance, where Michel lies in his tent and objects are hollow and alien, and the surroundings reduced to their contours: "Raindrops fell with a dull sound on the canvas; though they were inches from his face, they could not touch him here."[44] Or in *The Map and the Territory* where the artist Jed Martin seems to have taken on the artistic consequence of the fact that the world has become, in the words of Wallace, a map of the world.

What Wallace takes great care to emphasize in this particular context of the novel is the difference between fashionable anhedonia and clinical depression. He writes that "[i]t's of some interest that the lively arts of the millennial USA treat anhedonia and internal emptiness as hip and cool."[45] This attitude has little to do with clinical, pathological depression, with the "Bad Thing," or "It," as it is called here. Tellingly, this late passage in *Infinite Jest* accommodates a juxtaposition between Kate Gompert and Hal Incandenza; the youngest son of the Incandenza family, an extraordinary tennis talent and an incredibly bright student at school, who suffers terribly from anhedonia. Hal has not, the narrator states, "had a bona fide intensity-of-interior-life-type emotion since he was tiny; he finds terms like *joie* and *value* to be like so many variables in rarefied equations, and he can manipulate them well enough to satisfy everyone but himself that he's there, inside his own hull, as a human being – but in fact he's far more robotic than John Wayne [another tennis player at the academy]."[46] According to the narrator, Hal is too young to realize that anhedonia – a robotic existence, or a "numb emptiness" – is not the worst kind of depression: "Dead-eyed anhedonia is but a remora on the ventral flank of the true predator, the Great White Shark of pain. Authorities term this condition *clinical depression* or *involutional depression* or *unipolar dysphoria*."[47] What matters here is clearly not the terminological differences, but the affective differences between anhedonia and depression; the differences between how those feelings feel. The difference between the two – which seem and *almost* are identical – is the difference between a Euclidean and a non-Euclidean world, between a world that is nothing but geometry and a world that goes beyond geometry as we know it. It is the difference between "numb emptiness" and "The Great White Shark of pain;" between the affectlessness of abstraction and concrete, visceral pain; between cold forms that exist within the reach of the human imagination and an ungraspable black hole. It is in short the difference between an anhedonic who feels *nothing* and a depressed person who *feels* nothing.

Terror of the flames (depression vs. sadness)

It is here, in the latter condition, that suicide presents itself as a real danger. As Wallace writes in *Infinite Jest*:

The so-called "psychotically depressed" person who tries to kill herself doesn't do so out of quote "hopelessness" or any abstract conviction that life's assets and debits do not square. And surely not because death suddenly seems appealing. The person in whom *Its* invisible agony reaches a certain unendurable level will kill herself the same way a trapped person will eventually jump from the window of a burning high-rise. Make no mistake about people who leap from burning windows. Their terror of falling from a great height is still just as great as it would be for you or me standing speculatively at the same window just checking out the view; i.e. the fear of falling remains a constant. The variable here is the other terror, the fire's flames: when the flames get close enough, falling to death becomes the slightly less terrible of two terrors. It's not desiring the fall; it's terror of the flames. And yet nobody down on the sidewalk, looking up and yelling "Don't!" and "Hang on!", can understand the jump. Not really. You'd have to have personally been trapped and felt flames to really understand a terror way beyond falling.[48]

Earlier in her conversation with the doctor, Kate Gompert goes to great lengths to distinguish her depression from that of others, though she does not want to use the word depression: "I'm not one of the self-hating ones," she says.

> The type of like "I'm shit and the world'd be better off without poor me" type that says but also imagines what everybody'll say at their funeral. I have met types like that on wards. Poor-me-I-hate-me-punish-me-come-to-my-funeral. Then they show you a 20 X 25 glossy of their dead cat. It's all self pity bullshit. It's bullshit. I didn't have any special grudges. I didn't fail an exam or get dumped by anybody. All these types. Hurt themselves.[49]

She is not "just" sad, nor does she "just" want to hurt herself. She wants to kill herself. There is a big difference, she says, between the two, between wanting to hurt herself and kill herself. Suicide is precisely to be understood as an attempt *not to hurt anymore*: "It's not wanting to hurt myself it's wanting to *not hurt*."[50] This explains Kate Gompert's only wish: ECT or a sustained period of sedation, "a month on the outside."[51] Eventually, Kate Gompert does get more than a month on the outside: The plot of the novel involves a film called *Infinite Jest*,[52] so lethally entertaining that anyone watching it will never want do anything else for the rest of his or her life, leaving the (un)fortunate viewer in a vegetative zombie-like state. This is the destiny that awaits Kate, who in the end gets, not what she deserves, but what she wants: *A way out.*

The last thing we hear of Kate Gompert is that she sits in a bar with Remy Marathe, a member of the Canadian group of Wheelchair Assassins. In this scene Kate is drinking alcohol, on the verge of taking up her substance abuse again, and Marathe seems about to kidnap her and convince her to watch the film *Infinite Jest*. Before that, however, Marathe tells the strange story of how he lost his legs, became depressed, and met his wife (who has no skull) and basically *chose* to love her, at which point Kate declares: "Ramy, I don't think I'm like thinking this is a feel-better story at all."[53]

Depression and Bob Hope

To recapitulate so far: The depression of Kate Gompert in *Infinite Jest* is not quite sadness, not quite anxiety, not quite even anhedonia. However, there is a point of conjunction, especially insofar as the comparison between depression and anhedonia is concerned: A total lack of empathy. Despite the fact that depression does not amount to feeling nothing, it involves a loss of, not only the feeling *for* but, more radically, the feeling *of* the other. This is what the depressed person in the story of the same name and Kate Gompert have in common, despite the various differences between the two characters and the fictional frameworks within which they appear. They are both "incapable of empathy with any other living thing," they both suffer from an "anhedonic Inability To Identify," which is an "integral part of It," that is to say depression.[54]

Whether because of the endless narcissistic loops of the depressed consciousness – and consciousness of consciousness of consciousness – as in "The Depressed Person," or because of the sheer psychic and physical pain that wraps Kate Gompert in "*Its* black folds," it is in both cases impossible to attend to anything or anyone other than the self itself, which implies that they have also lost the future, if we follow Levinas' definition of the other as a figure of futurity. What separates the two, however, is that Kate is an addict; she is addicted to marijuana. After her hospitalization, Kate seeks admittance to the Ennet House Drug and Alcohol Recovery House. She smokes a lot of marijuana or "Bob Hope," as she calls it. She even, quite wittily and wittingly, suggests that her depression "maybe had to do with Hope," but the doctor does not understand the slang. She goes on to explain to him that she does "love it *so much*," that at times she smokes it excessively, but that she always stops after a given period of time. This is where "this *feeling* always starts creeping in," meaning the feeling of depression. This puzzles the doctor, since none of the clinical literature he has read "suggested any relation between unipolar episodes and withdrawal from cannabinoids."[55] Nonetheless, it is beyond any doubt that the convergence between addiction and depression is a constant theme in the novel.

Scene 3. "What looks like the cage's exit is actually the bars of the cage" (Joelle van Dyne and *Infinite Jest*)

Joelle van Dyne is excruciatingly alive and encaged, and in the director's lap can call up everything from all times. What will be the most self-involved of acts, self-cancelling, to lock oneself in Molly Notkin's bedroom or bath and get so high that she is going to fall down and stop breathing and turn blue and die, clutching her heart. No more back and forth [...] No more throwing the Material away and then half an hour later looting through the trash, no more all-fours scrutiny of the carpet in hopes of a piece of lint that looks enough like the Material to try to smoke [...] No more clutching her heart on a nightly basis. What looks like the cage's exit is actually the bars of the cage. The afternoon's meshes. The entrance says *EXIT*. There isn't an exit. The ultimate annular fusion: that of exhibit and its cage. Jim's own *Cage III: Free Show*. It is the cage that has entered *her*, somehow. The ingenuity of the whole thing is beyond her. The Fun has long since dropped off the Too Much. She's lost the ability to lie to herself about being able to quit, or even about enjoying it, still. It no longer delimits and fills the hole. It no longer delimits the hole. There's a certain smell to rain-wet veil. Something about the caller and the moon, saying the moon never looked away. Revolving and not. She had hurtled on back home on the night's final T and gone home and at least finally not turned her face away from the situation, the predicament that she didn't love it anymore she hated it and wanted to stop and also couldn't stop or imagine stopping or living without it. She had in any way done as they'd made Jim do near the end and admitted powerlessness over this cage, this unfree show, weeping, literally clutching her heart, smoking first the

Chore Boy-scrap she'd used to trap the vapors and form a smokable resin, then bits of the carpet and the acetate panties she'd filtered the solution through hours earlier, weeping and veilless and yarn-haired, like some grotesque clown, in all four mirrors of her little room's walls.[56]

In this scene a couple of hundred pages into *Infinite Jest*, Joelle Van Dyne prepares for her last taste of homemade freebase cocaine, which she smokes at a party at her friend Molly's apartment, before she admits to her drug problem and arrives at the doorstep of the Ennet House. Joelle van Dyne is a mysterious character. Using the pseudonym Madame Psychosis, she hosts a radio show popular among the tennis players at the Enfield Academy; she is also called PGOAT, an acronym denoting "prettiest girl of all time," and perhaps her stunning beauty is the reason she hides behind a veil, never letting anyone see her face (in the scene above, she is "veilless" because she is alone and her veil is "rain-wet"). Her own explanation is that she is in fact not pretty at all, but so disgustingly deformed that not only has she hidden behind a veil for quite some time, but has joined the UHID – the Union of the Hideously and Improbably Deformed. Moreover, she has been one of Orin Incandenza's lovers and acted in several of his father's experimental movies, including the infamous "Infinite Jest." What Joelle has in common with Kate and a lot of the other characters – besides painful experiences with anhedonic or depressive episodes – is an addiction to alcoholic or narcotic substances.

Too much fun

So, in this scene, what Joelle experiences is clearly not anhedonia, but it is not hedonia either. Rather, it seems like a case of an inability to do anything but to pursue *un*pleasure.[57] Her drug taking has gone from fun to unfun. She hates doing it and yet she cannot *not* do it. Now that Joelle has – supposedly – had enough, this is it: One last hit. She does not want to throw all her "Material away" and then regret it half an hour later, "no more all-fours scrutiny of the carpet in hopes of a piece of lint that looks enough like the Material to try to smoke."

The reason that Joelle began to smoke freebase cocaine in the first place is never unraveled. She did not have a rosy upbringing: Her own father fell in love with her, which appalled her mother/his wife so much that she eventually killed herself by sticking her arms into the garbage disposal. Yet, as always with Wallace, it is not tenable to place too much emphasis on these kinds of causal, etiological explanations. What remains clear is that addiction in Wallace's work always functions as a kind of (damaged) defense mechanism. As Andrew Weil makes clear at the outset of *The Natural Mind: A new way of looking at drugs and the higher consciousness* (1972) – a book that Wallace had read and kept in his private library – his "real interest is not drugs at all but consciousness."[58] In a certain sense the same goes for Wallace but with one decisive modification: The thing that Joelle and every other character in *Infinite Jest* looks for in the various substances they consume is not an *altered* consciousness, as in the psychedelic sixties, but a *suspended* consciousness. This is more in line with what Christopher Lasch briefly indicates in *The Culture of Narcissism*: "Anything to get his mind off his own mind."[59] With regard to my focus on psychopathology, depression and addiction often go hand in hand, and according to Alain Ehrenberg – whose general and persuasive idea is that "depression and addiction are what trace the outline of the individual at the end of the twentieth century"– addiction is a way to fill "the depressive void," a way "of compensating for it."[60]

In Wallace's work of course, addiction does not fill or erase the depressive void, nor do addictive habits help to take the drug addict's mind off his or her own mind. Rather, it intensifies obsessive thinking. Examples are legion. The narrator of *Infinite*

Jest, for example, claims "[t]hat most Substance-addicted people are also addicted to thinking, meaning they have a compulsive and unhealthy relationship with their own thinking [...] the cute Boston AA term for addictive-type thinking is: *Analysis-Paralysis*."[61] In *The Pale King* this is referred to as *obetrolling*: When the character Chris Fogle, a total "wastoid," does drugs he often experiences a heightening if not doubling of awareness, which is sometimes a nice experience, and sometimes not: "The awareness could sort of explode into a *hall of mirrors* of consciously felt sensations and thoughts and awareness of awareness of awareness of these."[62] This kind of stoned thinking has the negative effect of exploding awareness or consciousness into a "hall of mirrors," a metaphor that I have drawn attention to previously, not least at the end of the scene above: "All four mirrors of her little room's walls." The dominant image, though, is that of the cage, the unpleasant logic being that when Joelle tries to exit the cage, the exit is not an exit at all but simply leads deeper into the cage or into another cage; the thinking intensifies or the depression deepens. In any case, it only ever gets worse: "What looks like the cage's exit is actually the bars of the cage. The afternoon's meshes. The entrance says *EXIT*. There isn't an exit [...] The Fun has long since dropped off the Too Much."

Cruel optimism, slow death

Joelle's behavior is a perfect but painful example of what Lauren Berlant calls cruel optimism in her book of the same name. As Berlant writes: "Cruel optimism is the condition of maintaining an attachment to a significantly problematic object."[63] Or as Wallace himself writes in the essay "E Unibus Pluram: Television and US Fiction," where he confronts the intimate relation between addiction and technology, or television to be exact: The cruel thing about addiction is that "(1) it causes real problems for the addict, and (2) it offers itself as a relief from the very problems it causes."[64]

Joelle is indeed attached to a "significantly problematic object." Sadly, however, this problem is not hers alone: In the works of Wallace, and nowhere more so than in *Infinite Jest*, virtually every person is, in some sense, an addict. It seems that every optimistic attachment is a potential addiction. It is thus not only Kate Gompert or Joelle van Dyne who are tormented by drug habits, but every character in *Infinite Jest*. In his book *Machine-Age Comedy* Michael North points out that, whether we are talking about tennis or entertainment, marijuana or freebase cocaine, every activity follows the same recursive pattern: "An initial desire for fun, freedom, or even just change leads ironically to repetition, routine, machine dependency, and sometimes death… The term that Wallace uses for this process is *annularity*, a word he adopts from biology to denote a system that runs around in circles after its own tail."[65] This has its own cruel comedy. People running away from themselves toward themselves. Dogs chasing their own tails. In a significant scene from the movie *Infinite Jest,* the character played by Joelle meets a long lost friend as she walks through a revolving door, but as this person attempts to follow her inside, she tries to follow the person in question out, so the two of them end up going round and round in the revolving door.[66] *Das ist aber auch sehr komisch.* A circular comedy; a comedy of the circle. However, some of the comedy in *Infinite Jest* is more slapstick, for instance in a scene in which a man becomes completely addicted to M*A*S*H!

There is of course a difference between being addicted to M*A*S*H and to MDMA, but the logic of the process seems to be the same. In the vocabulary of Kierkegaard, what we see in this near-future world of capitalist consumption is that possibility is almost always already perverted into necessity. In more prosaic terms: Want turns into need, attachment into addiction, fun collapses into too much fun, and the pleasure principle is nothing more than the death-drive at its purest. This is addiction's sickness unto death in *Infinite Jest*. The character's attachments to their particular choice of drug are unhealthy and threaten their flourishing, and yet they cling to it, they want to yet cannot stop, even though it is killing them, not instantaneously, but slowly, ever so slowly: "A fuckin' livin' death, I tell you it's not being near alive, by the end I was undead, not alive, and I tell you the idea of dyin' was nothing compared to the idea of livin' like that for another five or ten years and only *then* dyin'," as one of the speakers says at an AA meeting, where it becomes clear that all the speakers' stories are alike. And the audience nods: "*boy* can they ever Identify."[67]

Wallace in Vegas: An addictive zone where man and machine are one

In his anatomy of addiction, Wallace is not merely interested in drugs – such as heroin, marijuana, Demerol, freebase cocaine – in a narrow sense. It would seem that a broader concept of drugs is needed to understand Wallace's work; one that, on the one hand, is not reducible to alcohol and narcotics, and on the other, is able to capture the simultaneous spiritual and technological dimensions of the relation between the subject and the desired object. The concept of "drugs" proposed by Félix Guattari is very useful in this regard: "We must begin by enlarging the definition of drugs. In my view, all the mechanisms producing a 'machinic' subjectivity, everything that contributes to provide a sensation of belonging to something, of being somewhere, along with the sensation of forgetting oneself, are 'drugs.'"[68]

Machines and technological apparatuses certainly play a central role in Wallace's works. For one, drug addicts watch enormous amounts of television and other forms of recorded entertainment in *Infinite Jest*. In the second chapter of the novel we meet Ken Erdedy who plans to spend "two straight days of heavy continuous smoking in front of the Inter-Lace viewer in his bedroom," the Inter-Lace viewer being the future version of television and the smoking marijuana. But it is not only drug addicts whom the Inter-Lace viewer is able to allure and bewitch, even if it is obviously not as lethal as the movie *Infinite Jest*. The general problem Wallace tries to address here is a society saturated with images and information, which the excessive footnotes in the book are supposed to reflect. Wallace is basically preoccupied by the pathological consequences – obsessive, compulsive or addictive behavior – of the daily overload of digital data. In the essay "E Unibus Pluram," Wallace contends that television has become our interior in such a way that it is hard to find a single human being whose attention, consciousness, sensibility, desire, perception and affectivity has not been captured and modulated by the technological apparatus of television. Wallace explores this idea in this essay, in *Infinite Jest*, as well as in *The Pale King*, where, for example, people are at one point described as "data processors." What is fabricated in the world of Wallace is, indeed, a "machinic" form of subjectivity – at the level of consciousness, desire, imagination and affect.

Empirical research supports this idea. In her book *Addiction by design. Machine Gambling in Las Vegas* (2012), American anthropologist Natasha Dow Schull details how gamblers do not play the slot machines to win; they play to play, to keep playing, to stay in the zone, in which a suspension of clock time and of chronological time is produced. She refers to an informant named Mollie, who states that her only goal is "to keep playing – to stay in that machine zone where nothing else matters."[69] Another informant, Lola, tells Dow Schull that she is "always hypnotized into *being* that machine [...] It's like playing against yourself: *You are the machine; the machine is you.*"[70] In this machine zone of addiction, subject and object, man and machine are one.

This corresponds to the more speculative thoughts that Guattari and his collaborator Gilles Deleuze advanced in *A Thousand Plateaus*, where they make a distinction between *social subjection* and *machinic enslavement*, their own example also being television: "One is subjected to TV insofar as one uses and consumes it," they write, but: "one is enslaved by TV as a human machine insofar as the television viewers are no longer consumers or users, not even subjects who supposedly "make" it, but intrinsic components, pieces, 'input' and 'output', feedback or recurrences that are no longer connected to the machine in such a way as to produce or use."[71]

In the process of machinic enslavement, a subject does not merely use an object as this distinction between subject and object no longer makes sense. A person caught up in this process is, as Maurizio Lazzarato comments, "*of a piece with* the machinic assemblages but he is also *torn to pieces* by it."[72]

The point here is that addiction in Wallace's work always operates as a form of machinic enslavement, which simultaneously pertains to something smaller and larger than the (addicted) individual or self. At one level, the individual – or dividual, as Deleuze and Guattari sometimes prefer to call it – is nothing but input and output, a small part in a gigantic statistical set of data based on algorithms of stunning sophistication. At another level, what is at stake is the innermost being of the individual, the neuronal networks and the minuscule movements of desire and affect. The zone of addiction is a prosthetic zone where one is "at piece with" the machine and yet "torn to pieces by it." It is a zone where all that matters is to keep playing, to stay in the *rhythm*.

What is to be done?

Although this scene took the character Joelle van Dyne and her addiction to drugs – culminating in her last hit of freebase cocaine – as its point of departure, it has been imperative, following Guattari's lead, to enlarge the definition of drugs. Television can function as a drug, as can tennis. The common denominator is a zone in which the distinction between subject and object, man and machine breaks down to the extent that it no longer makes any sense to say that the former is simply using the latter:

The entanglement is far deeper than that. And every attempt to escape the cage of addiction almost always leads deeper into the cage, and every attempt to escape a current situation and a present self by way of addiction – in order to suspend consciousness, stop thinking, numb the physical or psychic pain etc. – only seems to make matters worse: "What looks like the cage's exit is actually the bars of the cage."

What, then, is the solution? What does the cure entail? Is the only way out a form of disentanglement, an abandonment of attachments that are always on the verge of mutating into debilitating addictions? It does not seem so. Guattari seemed to offer a more viable approach in *The Anti-Œdipus Papers*, where he wrote, quite provocatively: "The criticism that consumption society deserves is that there are not enough things: we need more gadgets, and things and stuff, that we can box into other things, all this crap, a whole sexuality of gadgets. The Puritans still have too much control over consumer society!"[73] I do not mean to suggest that Wallace follows Guattari's schizoid thinking all the way – which he certainly did not – but that he acknowledges that there is, for all the cruel cul-de-sacs looming on the horizon, basically no going back. We cannot shrink away from the "things and stuff," that are, for better or worse, the texture of the world today. We cannot *not* believe, we cannot *not* attach ourselves to something: Everybody worships something or someone.[74] On the other hand it is obvious that Wallace did not want his characters – or his readers for that matter – to plunge heedlessly into the abyss of attachments. In reality, though, Wallace's concerns were more oriented toward people than toward things, toward the other rather than toward the object. However, Wallace cherished no illusions that relations between people could be easily established, let alone maintained. As he said in the interview with Larry McCaffery: "We all suffer alone in the real world. True empathy's impossible," although he then added: "But if a piece of fiction can allow us imaginatively to identify with a character's pain, we might then also more easily conceive of others identifying with their own. This is nourishing, redemptive; we become less alone inside. It might just be that simple."[75]

This is Wallace's ethico-spiritual "solution" to the problematic of depression, which resonates as argued with a problematic of addiction: A recovery of the other. That recovery necessitates an act of empathy, or in the idiom of the next scene, a work of love, though this has almost nothing to do with a mushy empathy, meant to unite self and other in simple and uncomplicated harmony.

Scene 4. Empathy as a radical work of love ("B.I. #20")

Q...

Yes and so in the anecdote there she is, blithely hitchhiking along the interstate, and on this particular day the fellow in the car that stops almost the moment she puts her thumb out happens to – she said she knew she'd made a mistake the moment she got in. The car. Just from what she called the energy field inside the car, she said, and that fear gripped her soul the moment she got in. And sure enough, the fellow in the car soon exits the highway and exits off into some kind of secluded area, which seems to be what psychotic sex criminals always do, you're always reading *secluded area* in all the accounts of quote *brutal sex slayings* and *grisly discoveries* of *unidentified remains* by a scout troop or amateur botanist, et cetera, common knowledge which you can be sure she was reviewing, horror-stricken, as the fellow began acting more and more creepy and psychotic even on the interstate and then soon exited into the first available secluded area.[76]

The loss of the other is the problem that Wallace presents and responds to in "The Depressed Person," in *Brief Interviews with Hideous Men* as a whole, in *Infinite Jest* and in the rest of his *oeuvre* for that matter. It is a problem of empathy, which, although rooted in the psychopathology of depression, has implications that go far beyond personal psychology. An ethical and cultural problematic is at work here as well. The terrain of the struggle begins with the recovery of the other. But in "The Depressed Person" the struggle is lost, if it is even begun in the first place. No risk of empathy is run here. Yet there is another story in the collection *Brief Interviews with Hideous Men*, "B.I. #20 12-96. New Haven CT" (hereafter abbreviated as "B.I. #20"), in which that risk *is* run and a possible remedy is offered. This is the story in which the ominous words quoted above appear. The story is the penultimate one in *Brief Interviews with Hideous Men,* and just like most of the other stories in this book, "B.I. #20" is an interview, presented in a classic Q&A-form, but with the important modification that all the questions have been left blank, making it impossible to determine what the answers are in fact answers *to.* It is in this context that the male interviewee is telling the anonymous interviewer a story about a woman he once met who told him a terrible story about a time she was hitchhiking and got into a car with a rapist and potential murderer and yet somehow escaped in the end. As should be evident from this brief introduction, "B.I. #20" has a number of rather complicated features such as the very framework of the story and multiple layers of storytelling, and the broader, societal question of a misogynic culture that it raises. What I wish to focus on is the moment where the woman saves her life. How does she do that, what happens, how are we, as readers, to interpret it, and what kind of model of empathy or love does the story provide?

New Age goo and the parable of the Good Samaritan

Sitting in the car with her future assailant, the female protagonist of the story feels instantly that something is terribly wrong. As the male interviewee tells the interviewer in *his* account of *her* account of the episode:

> Despite the terror she is somehow able to think quickly on her feet and thinks it through and determines that her only chance of surviving this encounter is to establish a quote connection with the quote soul of the sexual psychopath as he's driving them deeper into the woody secluded area looking for just the right spot to pull over and brutally have at her. That her objective is to focus very intently on the psychotic mulatto as

an ensouled and beautiful albeit tormented person in his own right instead of merely as a threat to her or a force of evil or the incarnation of her personal death.[77]

The rather cynical male interviewee knows that this might come across as one big, stupid cliché so he not only uses verbal quotation marks around words such as "connection" and "soul," but hastens to add, just to be on the safe side, that the interviewer needs to "try to bracket any New Age goo in the terminology and focus on the tactical strategy itself if you can because I'm well aware that what she is about to describe is nothing but a variant of the stale old Love Will Conquer All bromide."[78] And, miraculously, "the psychotic mulatto" does not kill the woman. He rapes her, so it is not as if nothing happens, but he does not kill her. She saves her life by this act of what the narrator calls "New Age goo," and later she (Sarah) meets the man (Eric) who is being interviewed in the story.

In the beginning his interest in her is purely sexual. She is, in his offensive formulation, "a quote Granola Cruncher, or post-Hippie, New Ager," who is sexy, not very intelligent and whose "prototypical Cruncher morphology" makes the closing of the erotic deal "almost criminally easy."[79] But when Sarah starts telling Eric the story everything changes; it turns out she is not only able to evoke empathy from the unnamed rapist but from Eric as well. However, the ending is rather ambivalent and disturbing, ending with Eric saying:

I believed she could save me. I know how this sounds, trust me. I know your type and I know what you're bound to ask. Ask it now. This is your chance. I felt she could save me I said. Ask me now. Say it. I stand here naked before you. Judge me, you chilly cunt. You dyke, you bitch, cooze, cunt, slut, gash. Happy now? All borne out? Be happy. I don't care. I knew she could. I knew I loved. End of story.[80]

Eric and the rapist are both unable to empathize, and they both have a noticeable tendency to treat women as "objects or dolls, *Its* and not *Thous*,"[81] which is precisely what for Simon Baron-Cohen is a sign of an erosion of empathy.[82]

It is in the context of this crisis of empathy that the parable of the Good Samaritan enters the picture. The parable (Luke 10:36) is the well-known story about a Jewish man who has been assaulted by robbers. A priest passes by without offering to help the poor man. A Levite also happens by, but he does not do anything either. It is finally a Samaritan – Jews and Samaritans ordinarily despised each other – who comes to the man's rescue. In the Bible, this is the story that Jesus tells to a Pharisee lawyer. But as Kierkegaard stresses in his breathtaking interpretation of the parable in *Works of Love* (*Kjerlighedens Gjerninger*, 1847) the Pharisee completely misunderstands the point of the story. The Pharisee thinks that the central question is, Who is my neighbor [*næste*]? That question, however, is deeply irrelevant, both to Jesus and to Kierkegaard. Instead of answering that question, Jesus, in Kierkegaard's re-telling, cunningly asks the Pharisee: "Which of these three seems to you to have been the neighbor to the man who had fallen among robbers?"[83] Formulating the question in that way now makes the Pharisee incapable of answering the question incorrectly. The neighbor to the man who had fallen among robbers is the Samaritan, the Pharisee says, whereupon Kierkegaard notes that

> the one to whom I have a duty is my neighbor, and when I fulfill my duty I show that I am a neighbor. Christ does not speak about knowing the neighbor but about becoming a neighbor oneself, about showing oneself to be a neighbor just as the Samaritan showed it by his mercy. By this he did not show that the assaulted man was his neighbor but that he was a neighbor of the one assaulted.[84]

Thus, the question is not "who is my neighbor" but "who is the neighbor of the other," which naturally will always be *me*. In Kierkegaard's account, this is the way the story unfolds and the recognition that is at stake. The assaulted man is not the Samaritan's neighbor. Rather, it is the other way around: the Samaritan is the neighbor of the assaulted man. That is what the Samaritan understands in stark contrast to the Levite and the priest. He is the only one truly able to love. But the act – or work – of love does not consist in the Samaritan loving his neighbor; instead, the love of the Samaritan entails presupposing the capacity for love in the neighbor. In that sense alone is love "upbuilding," (*opbyggelig*) as Kierkegaard formulates it: "*Love builds up by presupposing that love is present.*"[85]

One of Kierkegaard's aims is to distinguish love (of the neighbor) from compassion, pity and charity: "Ah, let the newspaper writers and tax collectors and the parish beadles talk about generosity and count and count," he writes satirically at one point. Also, as a figure, the neighbor is not identical with a loved one or a friend since, according to Kierkegaard, such persons are only versions or variations of the self itself: "In the beloved and the friend, it of course is not the neighbor who is loved, but the *other* I, or the first I once again, but more intensely."[86] The other in this context is transformed into a projection of the self – to an other I, a second I – and the so-called good deed is really an expression of self-love or even narcissism. As Kierkegaard observes, "Love for the neighbor cannot make me one with the neighbor in a unified self,"[87] as if the task of love merely consisted in walking around in the world, looking for lovable people. For Kierkegaard, the more cumbersome and important task is therefore to make oneself able to find any given object or person lovable, even to find "the un-lovable object lovable."[88] This radical act implies presupposing the capacity for love even, or especially, in a person who not only seems rather unlovable but also, and more importantly, utterly unloving. One might wonder if it is at all possible to love a person who is incapable of loving, and the answer is yes – except that it is precisely not to be taken as a question (am I able to love that person?) but as an imperative (you have to love that person!). Presupposing the capacity for love in the other is not about presupposing that this person *is* really capable of loving but that he or she *might* be able to; love is presupposed as a possibility, which means that love is also a matter of faith, of belief. You can never know for sure if the other is, ultimately, able to measure up to the infinite height of love. According to Kierkegaardian logic, what is certain is that you do not, under any circumstances, presuppose love in the other in order to be loved in return (as I detail below, love does not keep accounts).

Applying this reading of the Good Samaritan to a reading of Wallace's short story "B.I. #20," could it not be said that what Sarah does is precisely to presuppose the ability to love in the psychotic rapist, an unlovable object if ever there were one? She attempts to entertain the idea that the rapist's neighbor is actually *her* (which is not a case of Stockholm syndrome). She does not say, "You are my neighbor," but rather, "I am *your* neighbor." The difference is radical, since she does not make him into an object of her hippie-like, New-Age-ish love, but presupposes the capacity for love in him, thereby making *her* into the object of his potential love. More accurately, she makes herself into the thou that is so unfamiliar and frightening to the rapist. The radical and perverted gesture on her part is based on the premise that she is his neighbor, his other, not that he is her other, her neighbor. In this sense, Wallace – for all his thoughts on the subject – avoids the narcissistic and ultimately dehumanizing act of reducing the other, the rapist, to an object of Sarah's love. Instead he is made into a subject capable of love.

Admittedly, this is a disturbing and troublesome thought: a rape victim undertaking the work of loving her rapist. How could (a reading of) a story like this possibly not make its readers extremely uncomfortable? Is it not irresponsible and morally offensive? Does it not condone a culture of rape and excuse the sexual offenders? Not at all. The one thing that the story—as well as the book in which it is included—is attentive to is a culture of sexism and misogyny. Yet there is more to the story "B.I. #20" than the message that "men are pigs," "rape is bad," or "rape victims are traumatized." As Wallace remarks in the interview with Larry McCaffery, literature's job is not only to "comfort the disturbed"; it is also to "disturb the comfortable," and it is the latter dimension I am highlighting here.[89] To avoid any misunderstandings, I am emphatically *not* suggesting that Wallace condones a misogynistic rape culture (quite the contrary in fact); or that he is insensitive toward the trauma of rape victims. Nor that Wallace is advocating that these victims should simply learn to love their offenders. What I *am* claiming is that this story reveals the radical nature of empathy and love, and the impossible, almost absurd work it requires (not entirely unlike the story of Abraham and Isaac, a story that only the most careless readers would interpret as a defense of filicide, or as a call for fathers to sacrifice their sons). The rape story is not to be read as Wallace's universal model of empathy – as if an ethical or a political praxis could be derived from the transposition of love as a reaction to rape – but as a brutal scene where one's (the character's as well as the reader's) capacity for love and empathy is pushed to the extreme. So if it is indeed a test of empathy – a test of "the boundaries of our willingness to 'empathize'" as Marshall Boswell puts it[90] – then it is precisely a test of our ability to presuppose the capacity for empathy in the other, that is, the hideous man. Only in this sense does love in fact "Conquer All."

The relation between self and other is not characterized by a reciprocal altruism, whereby I do something for you *now* in expectation that you will return the favor *in the future.* In *Works of Love* Kierkegaard even explicitly writes that love transcends every form of "bookkeeping arrangement."[91] Love is a gift that one gives without expecting something in return, without any demand for profit or repayment. True love has never heard of the principle *quid pro quo*; it knows no numbers. Paradoxically, in an act of love, it is the giver and not the receiver who puts himself in debt. In this regard Kierkegaard speaks of an "infinite debt" which defies any kind of arithmetical calculation.

This thought is not only echoed in Wallace's idea of infinity, as presented both in *Infinite Jest* and *Everything and More,* where two varieties of infinity are distinguished; a "good" one like that proposed by Kierkegaard, and a "bad" one like that referred to throughout Wallace's work as a vicious infinite regress. It also ties in with the discourse of Alcoholics Anonymous and Narcotics Anonymous in *Infinite Jest,* adhering to the clichés of taking it one day at a time and living completely in the moment: "It's a gift, the Now: it's AA's real gift; it's no accident they call it *The Present.*"[92] The present – or what Kierkegaard conceptualizes as Øieblikket (*Augenblick* in German) – is a present, a gift, but it is not a gift one receives; it is rather something one gives, something one passes to an other, placing oneself in a situation of *infinite debt.* The difficult task, then, is how to stay in debt to the other. That is, what Kierkegaard calls the "element" of love. The decisive condition is that one refrains from engaging in any accounting measures, that one avoids doing "bookkeeping" and that one leaves all judgments and comparisons behind. "Beware of comparison!" Kierkegaard cautions the reader of *Works of Love,*[93] a warning one could have wished that the protagonist of "The Depressed Person" could have known and taken note of, for what is her mental apparatus but one big machine of comparison? Is she not continuously "working on the treadmill of comparison" that Kierkegaard describes so well?[94] One of the remarkable symptoms of her depressive condition is that she constantly compares her cheerless life with the vibrating, active and meaningful lives that she, unjustly and erroneously, imagines the members of her support system lead. In the words of Kierkegaard, she cannot help "counting and weighing," as she is caught in the compulsive refrain of comparison.

It is the belief and not the god that counts

The fact that empathy—which, as I have just argued, is to be taken as synonymous to an extent with the Kierkegaardian notion of love that emerges in his reading of the Good Samaritan—is an inherently "therapeutic" project for Wallace is strikingly clear in the way Alcoholics Anonymous and Narcotics Anonymous operate in *Infinite Jest*. They are examples of the novel's "technologies of the self" (along with the Assassins en Fauteuils Roulants and Enfield Tennis Academy, i.e. terrorism and tennis), providing places for addicts to listen to the stories of other addicts without ever judging or comparing.[95] A place for empathy. "Empathy, in Boston AA, is called Identification," the narrator of the novel states, which means that the participants, particularly newcomers, are encouraged to "Identify instead of Compare. Again, *Identify* means empathize."[96] These sentences are easy to misunderstand and trivialize, but the procedure of identifying and empathizing is precisely not about comparing, as Kierkegaard reminds us, nor about erasing the otherness of the other, so that the other merely becomes a version or an alter ego of the I. "The relationship with the other," as Levinas notes, "is not an idyllic and harmonious relationship of communion, or a sympathy through which we put ourselves in the other's place; we recognize the other as resembling us, but exterior to us; the relationship with the other is a relationship with a Mystery."[97]

Where Wallace parts ways with both Kierkegaard – and Levinas – is in his emphasis on the communal quality of Alcoholics Anonymous and Narcotics Anonymous. This idea brings me back to Karl Jaspers, for whom the question of belief and faith is a practical, collective one. In his *General Psychopathology*, Jaspers argues that psychotherapy itself "must be set within a frame of common beliefs and values" if it is to have any chance of bringing about "collaboration of doctor and patient in a mutual philosophical faith."[98] This form of belief, however, cannot be reduced to any therapeutic relation; rather, it depends upon belief and trust in other people. *"Sharing in something objective*—whether symbols, a faith, the accepted philosophy of some group—is a necessary condition for any profound cohesion among men," Jasper argues, adding that "many modern psychotherapists labour under the illusion that, when faced with neuroses and personality disorders, the highest possible expectation is realisation of the patient's own self."[99] Belief, in other words, is a shared enterprise.

At the same time, it is crucial to remember that, like Jaspers, most of the characters in Wallace's work, not to mention Wallace himself, remain skeptics. They are people who do not have any faith to begin with, for whom faith and belief are strenuous, tedious tasks that require, for all their quotidian qualities, a leap of faith in the sense deployed by Kierkegaard, who not only stressed the absurdity of this leap but fought hard to maintain belief in his own private life. What we have here is belief without belief, maybe even a belief against belief, a kind of faith of the faithless. "It is the belief and not the god that counts," the poet Wallace Stevens writes in the text Adagia. "The final belief is to believe in a fiction, which you know to be a fiction, there being nothing else. The exquisite truth is to know that it is a fiction and that you believe it willingly."[100]

The concept of *fiction* is important here. It ought to be quite clear by this point that the preceding considerations have some implications for a rethinking of the relationship between fiction and empathy in Wallace's work. If depression can, and indeed must, be understood as a lack of empathy, and if fiction is understood as an exercise in empathy, then fiction and "therapy" are consequently brought into an intimate and affirmative affiliation with one another: it is here, potentially, that other rhythms can arise and a restoration of empathy take place.

Wallace's oeuvre is saturated with scenes of storytelling. The community of Alcoholics Anonymous and Narcotics Anonymous in *Infinite Jest* is a case in point: the sharing of stories forms the foundation of every meeting and every group. The story "B.I. #20" is evidently another. The story features a nameless and implicit narrator who tells a story to the reader about a man, the interviewee, who tells a story to his interviewer, about a story a woman told him, about a time when she was raped and nearly killed. In these multiple layers of fiction, what is key is the concrete situation of narrating and listening. To be more precise, the emphasis is not so much on the narrator as on the listener in Wallace's works. This is the case in "B.I. #20," in the posthumous *The Pale King* whose protagonist Shane Drinion is capable of listening with so much focus and concentration that he literally elevates from his chair, and in *Infinite Jest* in which the deformed Mario is the ultimate listener, as his brother Hal knows all too well: "And maybe that's the key. Maybe then whatever's said to you is so completely believed by you that, what, *it becomes sort of true in transit*. Flies through the air toward you and reverses its spin and hits you true, however mendaciously it comes off the other person's stick," says Hal to Mario.[101]

Again, it is rather obvious that the focus is less on the self, on the Samaritan or on the narrating figure than on the other, the neighbor, the listener. One might even say that the "you" is primary to the "I" in Wallace's literature. But his work does not train our capacity for empathy and our moral imagination by inviting or forcing us as readers to put ourselves in another person's shoes for a while. Unlike, for example, Martha Nussbaum, who has commented extensively on the relation between literature and empathy and who speaks of a moral judgment based on an "empathic imagining," i.e. on "experiencing what happens to them [the characters] as if from their point of view,"[102] the key is not that the reader is or becomes able to empathize in order to arrive at the point at which a moral judgment can be made. It is precisely the act of comparison and judgment that we need to leave behind; to paraphrase Hegel's *Philosophy of Right,* Wallace's stories constitute no court of judgment. The task is to listen, or as *Infinite Jest* puts it, the task is "I.D.ing without effort. There's no judgment."[103] Only in this way is fiction able to achieve a therapeutic and ethical function, reconstructing the relation to the other that has been lost or damaged in depression. Fiction can, in the words of Franco "Bifo" Berardi, make possible a different and less obsessive refrain than that of depression; it can create a change in the rhythms of life, generate another set of "relations between what you believe and what you believed before," to quote the lines from *Brief Interviews with Hideous Men* one last time. And sometimes it can or does not, as in "The Depressed Person," where the protagonist's narcissistic narration leaves no room for listening (perhaps this means that the story gives expression to an even stronger and more radical version of Kierkegaard's concept of love, since all the work needs to be done by the reader in relation to a totally unlovable, depressed protagonist, given that the story itself makes no attempt to love her).

At issue here are not only the discrete scenes and situations in Wallace's body of work but also, and perhaps above all, what the works themselves do, what they practice and produce. It stands to reason that the relation between speaker and listener *in* the respective stories reflects the relation between narrator or writer and reader *of* the stories. Here too, it is the case that whatever is said and told only becomes "true in transit." In Wallace's fiction, the act of storytelling represents not only the possibility of empathy, love, and a restoration of the other but, more strongly, a precondition. It bears repeating that it is not a matter of who my neighbor is but who the neighbor of the other is. Being able to love an unlovable object (and the men in *Brief Interviews with Hideous Men* are most certainly unlovable) is imperative, but it can only be done if I presuppose the capacity for empathy and love in the other, not through exposing or subjecting him or her to my overwhelming empathy, compassionate love, or moral judgment. Wallace's fiction is an "upbuilding" form of literature, which is what the story "B.I. #20" shows more than any other piece by Wallace: It builds up love and empathy by presupposing that love and empathy are present in the other, even, and especially, when love and empathy are clearly not there at all. This ethical and even spiritual project in a literary form is animated and made necessary by the pathological problem of depression. Whether it is translatable into a political project, or capable of assuming a form and function that goes beyond the relatively limited sphere of writer and reader, or a community of ex-addicts, is a question for another occasion.

One-two-three paradoxes (Threshold)

What the first two scenes of this chapter have shown regarding the problem of depression is that, whether the problem and pathology are related to a narcissistic self-consciousness and self-absorption, as is the case for the female protagonist in "The Depressed Person," or to a sheer physical and mental pain, as is the case for Kate Gompert in *Infinite Jest*, the result is the same: A loss of empathy, a loss of the other as a category of futurity. In spite of the disparate nature of the two stories, with regard to content and form, this is the point of convergence characteristic of the experience of depression in Wallace's works: "A person in such a state is incapable of empathy with any other living thing."[104]

This is the problem of depression that Wallace presents and responds to. As we have seen in scene three, it is a problem that is inseparable from a more general and thoroughly American problem of addiction. What is articulated in Wallace's work in general, and in *Infinite Jest* in particular, is that addiction to drugs is the mirror image of depression. Within the framework of this book, depression and addiction mirror each other in that a total *isolation* from the other – person or object – is at work in depression, whereas in addiction the issue is one of total *immersion*. While there is an obvious contrast between depression and addiction – isolation vs. immersion, detachment vs. attachment – and while the two meanings can thus be seen as opposed to each other, this may not necessarily be so. Both can be said, in Wallace, to form part of the same repetitive circle, the same loop of reflection, the same form of bad infinity, the same version of vicious infinite regress, which in the end (if not immediately) leads to a devastating loss of the future. And both lose the other, though from opposite directions so to speak. That is the pathological figure as Wallace exposes it, but there is another figure, one that contains the possibility for change, and of a therapeutic cure. This is the straight line that breaks open the circle and leads where, exactly? Into the unknown. It can lead to death and suicide, but it can lead to redemption, reparation and recovery too, it can lead to a restoration of the being of the other. As evidenced in scene four of this chapter a leap of faith is required, a radical work of love, a transcendent trajectory that disrupts the circular rhythm of pure pathology.

But is this leap of faith even possible for the depressed person, given that (s)he is depressed? Is there not something paradoxical in this demand? Kierkegaard notes this very paradox in *Works of Love*: "Humanly speaking, it is indeed most strange, almost like mockery, to say to the despairing person that he shall do that which was his sole desire but the impossibility of which brings him to despair. Is any other evidence needed that the love commandment is of divine origin!"[105] The paradox is: How do you reach out to and for the other when the other is that which cannot be reached? (first paradox).

Another question emerges though: How can we know that the restoration of the other does not cause a heightened rather than diminished risk of violence? How would we ensure that a new attachment does not mutate into a new addiction, that optimism does not become cruel, that surrender of the self to something bigger than the self does not lead to totalitarianism, or a new narcissism? How do we know that the self is not selfish in its utter selflessness, that the exit from the cage of depression does not lead deeper into the cage? The point is, we would not know, nor could we ever know. This is, so to speak, the basic condition of faith. There is only one resolution, which is that there is no resolution (second paradox).

In any case, it ought to be clear by now that Wallace was a deeply spiritual writer. He thought it was time to take seriously such questions of depression, addiction and belief, of therapy and art. His books show how what one attaches oneself to is of the greatest and gravest importance. As the character Remy Marathe says in *Infinite Jest:* "Our attachments are our temple, what we worship, no? What we give ourselves to, what we invest with faith," adding, "Choose with care. You are what you love. No?"[106] We cannot *not* believe in something. Everybody worships, as Wallaces states in *This is Water*. Emancipation in his work is clearly not a Pinocchean endeavor, it does not equal an autonomous state without strings. Rather, it entails being well attached to the other: "That is real freedom."[107] And where does this leave fiction? Is literature to be understood as spiritual therapy?

Susan Sontag opened her text "The Aesthetics of Silence" from 1967 with the words: "Every era has to reinvent the project of 'spirituality' for itself,"[108] but what would that mean in the case of Wallace? Perhaps the production of a literature that would not be content with – cynically and ironically, *à la* Easton Ellis or Houellebecq – exposing and criticizing the world as it is, and that would not be reducible to "a mordant deadpan commentary on the badness of everything." A literature based on the recognition that critique and negativity is not, in itself, enough. This was what William James realized and pointed out perceptively more than 100 years ago. In *Varieties of Religious Experience* – a book that Wallace had read and appropriated in his writing on depression – the chapter on the sick souls is preceded by a chapter on the mind-cure movement, also known as New Thought. Here James records a significant shift in society: The replacement of traditional religious institutions and movements by other forms of therapeutic relief and redemption. As he writes: "The mind-cure with its gospel of healthy-mindedness has come as a revelation to many whose hearts the church of Christianity had left hardened."[109] According to James the movement is based on principles of health, happiness and optimism, and the conviction that thoughts are things, implying that what matters most is not objective reality but subjective thoughts, perceptions and feelings pertaining to this reality. In other words: If one changes one's mental apparatus, then one can change reality – which bears striking resemblance to the jargon of contemporary self-help books, positive psychology and cognitive therapy, where happiness is a matter of personal choice and the right attitude. Yet, instead of simply dismissing this movement out of hand, James took it seriously and treated it as "a genuine religion." As a consequence, anyone interested in offering an alternative to this "genuine religion" must acknowledge the need for relief for sick souls and be prepared to offer an equally appealing alternative if one wishes to have any effect at all: "No prophet can claim to bring a final message unless he says things that will have a sound of reality in the ears of the victims [...] But the deliverance must come in as strong a form as the complaint."[110] However, in Wallace's writing the deliverance that James talks about is often denied to the very characters that need it the most. There is, for instance, no "deliverance" for the depressed person from the story of the same name, nor is there one for Kate Gompert in *Infinite Jest*, though of course Wallace's task as a writer is not to ensure a happy ending for each and every one of his characters. One can almost hear them whispering to themselves, quoting Kafka: Oh, there is hope, only not for us (third paradox).

Chapter 3

Shooting the ambulance? – Claire Fontaine

Introduction

Even the name is a ready-made. Claire Fontaine is a French company that specializes in stationery, but since 2004 it has also been the name of a duo formed by the Italian artist Fulvia Carnevale and the British artist James Thornhill.[1] The artist Claire Fontaine not only makes ready-made art, she is a ready-made artist who, practicing a radical, uncompromising avant-garde art of a conceptual and minimalist disposition, has renounced on the idea of a creative, artistic and romantic subject. Within the scene of contemporary art, Claire Fontaine is one of the artists who have worked in the most concentrated and consistent way with the problem of depression. But Claire Fontaine has moved far beyond the domain of clinical depression: There is no phenomenological experience of depression, no representation of a depressed subjectivity. In their work, depression is always already political and must be understood in relation to its real basis in social conflicts within a neoliberal economy of debt and financial speculation.

In her art Claire Fontaine thus responds to depression as a pertinent contemporary problem, just as we have seen Michel Houellebecq and David Foster Wallace do. However, whereas Houellebecq's ontological/technological response pertains to something other than being, and Wallace's ethical/spiritual response pertains to the being of the other, Claire Fontaine's response takes a radically different form. Indeed, from her point of view, Houllebecq's response is probably to be condemned for being reactionary, and Wallace's for being too humanistic and apolitical. For Claire Fontaine, depression is – or can be – seen as a political action, a human strike, which becomes a contemporary and psychopathological form of strike. Neoliberal capitalism, in her understanding, forms a totality that does not only have an effect on society at a structural level or on people at an individual level, but encroaches on social relations, feelings and the very being of human beings. The strike must therefore interact at all those levels as well, and assume a total character. The human strike is – as Claire Fontaine herself articulates it in the text "Human Strike Within the Field of Libidinal Economy" – "a type of strike that involves the whole of life and not only its professional side, that acknowledges exploitation in all the domains and not only at work."[2] Accordingly, the human strike is not about ceasing to work for the purpose of improving working conditions, for instance. In fact, the human strike is purely and exclusively a process of the present and has no future objectives; it is not a means to an end but pure means – an idea Claire Fontaine borrows from Giorgio Agamben.

It should be said that there is something strange about some, if not most of Claire Fontaine's works. Powerful and dramatic as they certainly are, they do not really appeal to analytical inquiry; something about them seems to ward off a detailed and meticulous close reading.[3] Yet, scene one will examine the critique of the political economy that Claire Fontaine unfolds in their video installation *P.I.G.S* from 2011. The prismatic vantage point for this scene is the concept of debt. As I will point out in more detail below there is an intimate relation between the current debt regime and neoliberal capitalism. Of particular interest will be the implications of debt on the level of temporality and subjectivity. Scene two and scene three then begin to hone in on depression. Using the ready-made work *Untitled (The Invisible Hand)* from 2011 as an object of analysis and an occasion for reflection, scene two concentrates on the question of temporality, while scene three attends to the question of subjectivity in Claire Fontaine's video work *Untitled (Why your psychology sucks)* from 2015, which offers a stark yet rather comical critique of the self-help ideology. Scene four then goes on to address the question of how depression can be seen as a human strike in the work and world of Claire Fontaine and if depression should perhaps be seen as a "solution" to the contemporary crisis rather than as "symptom" of it? In which case, the question becomes: How valid and tenable is this solution, if it is a solution at all? And can art really be or become a strike in the proper sense of the term?

Such questions animate this chapter, the structure of which follows, in the order given, three key concepts: Debt, depression, strike. Or, to put it in slightly different and definitely cruder terms: Problem, symptom, cure.

Scene 1. Burning P.I.G.S (Debt in the neoliberal era)

A white wall and thousands of matches. This is what Claire Fontaine's installation video *P.I.G.S* consists of, at least at the outset. The matchsticks are placed in the wall in the form of maps of Portugal, Italy, Greece and Spain; the countries that make up the so-called PIGS at the periphery of the Euro zone (sometimes Ireland receives the "honor" of being included in this group, transforming PIGS to PIIGS). The derogatory term denotes the nation-states that suffer the most under the current debt crisis. Southern Europe is – so to speak – in flames, which is what the work by Claire Fontaine aims to show in a very concrete way. In the video, a hooded man enters the frame with a flamethrower in his hand. He approaches the western part of the map and ignites Portugal and Spain, then Italy and finally Greece. Then he leaves. The image is nothing but fire and there is no sound except for the crackling wood and the soaring flames, which last until everything is burned down to an incinerated color and only a glowing red is visible at the edges of each ash-defined country. Parts of the wall have by now also been smeared black by the fire and a dark smoke becomes ever-more intense, rising upward and clouding most of the screen. At some point an alarm goes off, possibly a fire alarm. After close to 10 minutes, the video ends. *In girum imus nocte et consumimur igni...*

Flames of debt in Southern Europe

Every single one of Claire Fontaine's works interrogates the contemporary condition, the current crisis, or rather, plural crises. The work "Gather in multiple groups" (2011) is a comment on Occupy, re-appropriating various statements from a flier found in Zuccotti Park in New York and spray painting them onto a canvas. The ongoing series "Foreigners Everywhere," comprising neon signs that utter the sentence "Foreigners Everywhere" in various languages, is a comment on the so-called refugee crisis. "P.I.G.S" unearths the disastrous debt situation in the southern part of the Euro zone.

Addressing the economic system in place – and in crisis – today, activist and sociologist Andrew Ross, who has participated in Occupy and in particular the offshoot movement "Strike Debt," has developed the concept of a *creditocracy*. In his book of the same name Ross is concerned with the seemingly endless accumulation of debt, whether in relation to housing, student or medical loans. These loans are, according to Ross, not by-products of the economic and financial system, but absolutely necessary for this system to function, and equally for nation-states to maintain and increase their respective GDP-growth, if indeed they have growth at all.[4] A similar analysis is made by the anthropologist David Graeber, whose bestseller *Debt – the first 5000 years,* makes the case that debt is at the center of political life in an unprecedented way, to the extent that "US household debt is now estimated at on average 130 percent of income."[5] By the same token sociologist Wolfgang Streeck has detailed how the state has gradually moved from being a tax state to a debt state, concluding that "the present financial, fiscal and economic crisis is the end point so far of the long neoliberal transformation of postwar capitalism."[6] It is indeed "a crisis that has a long story and, in all likelihood, a long future."[7] Or as Kojin Karatani writes in *Transcritique*: "Credit and crisis go hand in hand."[8]

Although it is not as though debt was not a problem before the crisis of 2008 – given both that the relation between debtor and creditor is, in a sense, as old as human kind and that the transition toward a financialized economy of debt has been at least 4 or 5 decades in the making – it has surely become an ever-more pertinent problem after the crisis, to say nothing of the role that the infamous collateralized debt obligations and credit default swaps played in the excessive acts of financial speculation during the years leading up to it. In less than 10 years, levels of debt have simply exploded. In October 2016, the Fiscal Monitor of the IMF issued a report with the unbelievably commonsensical title "Debt. Use It Wisely." The report states that "at 225 percent of world GDP, the global debt of the nonfinancial sector—comprising the general government, households, and nonfinancial firms—is currently at an all-time high." That global debt is at "an all-time high" is not that surprising, but 225 percent of world GDP is still a very high number, amounting to roughly $152 trillion. An accompanying blog post on IMFblog – the International Monetary Fund's global economy forum – even emphasizes that "the picture is not pretty."[9]

Obviously, debt is distributed unequally, along axes of race, gender, class etc. The report by IMF observes "there is considerable heterogeneity, as not all countries are in the same phase of the debt cycle, nor do they face the same risks," to which the accompanying blog post adds that not "all countries are in the same boat." Some people and some countries carry a greater burden than others. For instance, it is well known that Southern Europe suffered the hardest blow under and after the economic crisis, and has still not recovered. The IMF-report includes a table of the general government debt-to-GDP ratio in the so-called advanced economies, which shows the amount of a country's total gross government debt as a percentage of its GDP, indicating how healthy and sustainable each economy is. Greece, Italy, Portugal and Spain are placed at the very bottom – or top, depending on how one looks at it – among European countries. The general government gross debt for Greece was thus 183.4 percent of its GDP in 2016, compared with 103.1 percent in 2007; for Italy, it was 133.2 percent in 2016, versus 99.8 percent in 2007; for Portugal 128.4 percent, versus 68.4 percent; and for Spain 101.5 percent, versus 35.5 percent. It is not a pretty picture at all.[10]

It should come as little surprise, then, that Claire Fontaine

have chosen these four countries to be set on fire in the work
P.I.G.S., since they are, in a sense, already in flames (and let it
be noted in passing that a sector of the economy goes by the
acronym FIRE, which stands for Finance, Insurance and Real
Estate). Of course, in this work Claire Fontaine is not interested
merely in the fiscal policy of Southern Europe. The artist duo
is not content with simply mapping out the socio-political
structure in an abstract yet dramatic fashion; what good would
that do? *P.I.G.S* moves beyond pure description; it entails a
call to action, a prescriptive encouragement. As argued by the
curators for the 4th Thessaloniki Biennale of Contemporary Art
(2013–2014), which featured *P.I.G.S*, the fire in the work, "which
represents at present time merely the destructive violence of the
financial crisis, could be the one of a revolution, burning the
debt before people get burned."[11] Burning the debt was indeed
part of the strategy of the Strike Debt movement of Occupy.
Under the slogans "Debt resistance for the 99%" and "You are
not a loan," this movement has produced *The Debt Resisters'
Operations Manual*, launched the Rolling Jubilee – "a Strike Debt
project that buys debt for pennies on the dollar, but instead of
collecting it, abolishes it," the homepage explains – and staged
several debt burnings in San Francisco, New York and elsewhere.
Clare Fontaine clearly alludes to such movements and moments
in *P.I.G.S*. One of their other works, *Untitled (Sell Your Debt)*, is
a white, blue and red neon sign saying "Sell your debt," which
for one exhibition was accompanied by *burnt/unburnt*, a work
almost identical to *P.I.G.S*, except the matches form a map of the
US.

The first point to take away from this is that Claire Fontaine's
work is as prescriptive as it is descriptive. Andrew Culp and
Ricky Crano observe in an interview with Claire Fontaine that
the works the artist duo produce (coins furnished with steel box-
cutter blades, books transformed into brickbats etc.) are, on the
one hand, "commodities in an art world ruled by collectors and

deals" and on the other objects "turned into tools for sabotage."[12] According to Culp and Crano the question thus posed by the art of Claire Fontaine "is not 'What does it mean?' nor 'What can we do with it?' but 'What do we want to do?' and, even more important, 'How is it that we, good consumers of capitalist art that we are, come to repress those desires?'"[13]

The second is that though there is a certain resonance between works such as *P.I.G.S* and *Untitled (Sell Your Debt)*, and the Strike Debt movement of Occupy, there is also a crucial difference. There is no direct action in Claire Fontaine's works, no catharsis or potent multitude that rises to face and rebel against an unjust economic system, be it in the southern European crisis countries or in the major cities of the US. Rather, there is a sense of impotence in their works, which makes for a strange kind of avant-garde art.[14] As such, the (historical) avant-garde entailed a certain futurism typical of the twentieth century. In itself it was a temporal figure; a figure of the future, a frontrunner and a vanguard. Claire Fontaine is no such thing, though she places herself in the avant-garde tradition, using the methods of re-appropriation, ready-made, and détournement that Marcel Duchamp, the Situationists and many others developed and practiced. Claire Fontaine is an avant-garde without any vanguard, an avant-garde that has, paradoxically, no revolutionary belief in the future, the one thing that defined the avant-gardism of yesterday. In that sense Claire Fontaine is a totally exhausted, if not downright depressed avant-garde. All that remains are gestures, reduced to their formal skeleton; a dried-up didacticism: "In our lifetime, we've only had the chance to see the effects of the Situationalist religion, this purism and extreme moralism that doesn't help to change anything at all. We needed to make fun of such a paradoxical position. But today, maybe it's like shooting the ambulance."[15] What Claire Fontaine tries to do in general is "to transcribe symptoms of the crisis, visually, and conceptually,"[16] and depression is certainly one of those topical symptoms – but so is art.

The third point is that the crisis, the artistic anatomy of which they perform, is not only an economic crisis. In their eyes, it is a crisis of subjectivity, affectivity and temporality as well.

Debt and depression ("I am not committing suicide. They are killing me")

In the book *The Making of the Indebted Man. An essay on the Neoliberal Condition,* Maurizio Lazzarato presents two fundamental hypotheses about debt. 1) Debt is the paradigm of the neoliberal economy of today. 2) Debt does not only amount to a structural question of the neoliberal economy. As for this second hypothesis – the first is accepted without further ado – Lazzarato makes clear that debt or credit produces a specific trinity of subjectivity, morality and temporality.[17] He draws for this idea upon Nietzsche, who in On *the Genealogy of Morality* attached great importance to the twofold meaning of *Schuld,* connoting both economic indebtedness and moral guilt.[18] Moreover, Nietzsche states that debt always assumes the form of a promise that for the parties involved, implies not only a "memory of the future" but makes the subject responsible for his or her own future. The indebted subject, as someone who makes a promise, becomes "answerable for his own *future!*" Nietzsche emphatically writes, adding that this "is precisely what constitutes the long history of the origins of responsibility."[19] In this sense, through the combination of responsibilization and futurity, the credit-relation pertains to the very being of indebted man, insofar as what is affected is the "morality of the debtor, his mode of existence (his 'ethos')," in the words of Lazzarato.[20]

Needless to say, the temporal relation of credit is first and foremost a relation of futurity; a relation to the future. As Lazzarato also notes, debt is based on the promise of a future installment or reimbursement, and the debt economy as a whole "is an economy that requires a subject capable of accounting for himself *as a future subject,* a subject capable of promising and keeping a promise, a subject that works on the self."[21] In short, debt in the neoliberal era cannot be reduced to a question of economic structures alone. As argued by Lazzarato and Nietzsche, the implications of debt on human subjectivity are quite severe. It could even be stipulated that a specific pathological structure is created in a situation like the present. If the goal of the preceding paragraphs has been to indicate an almost intrinsic relation between capitalism and credit, between what Lazzarato calls the neoliberal condition and the indebted man, then what remains to be attended to is the relation between debt and depression, as depression is the predominant pathology within this historical formation.

Following in the wake of the current economic crisis, a plethora of studies have looked into the psychological consequences of debt. In the article "Debt and Depression: Causal Links and Social Norm Effects," economist John Gathergood shows that people awash in a sea of debt experience and exhibit a variety of mental problems, including depression.[22] By all accounts, it seems that being indebted can, and indeed does, lead to an increased risk not only of depression but also suicide. This is the point of interest for the article "Personal debt and suicidal ideation," where the authors, a group of mental health scientists, document that "those in debt were twice as likely to think about suicide after controlling for sociodemographic, economic, social and lifestyle factors."[23] And in *The Body Economic: Why Austerity Kills,* David Stuckler and Sanjay Basu have conducted an epidemiological research project, using statistics and large-scale data sets to understand health epidemics and economy, which demonstrates that austerity policies – rather than recession as such – have terrible, often deadly, consequences for the state of public and private health. At one point in their book Stuckler and Basu refer to a particular study of Americans over the age of 50 which found "that between 2006 and 2008, people who fell behind on their mortgage payments were about nine times more likely to develop depressive symptoms."[24] Their bleak conclusion is that austerity not only hurts, but kills, exemplified by the tragic case of the Greek Dimitris Christoulas, who on April 4, 2012, "put a gun to his head in front of the Greek parliament and declared: 'I am not committing suicide. They are killing me.' Then he pulled the trigger."[25]

This example could have been taken directly from Claire Fontaine's portfolio. In 2010, they made a video called *Suicide Stack*, which revolves around the software engineer Joseph Stack who in February 2010 flew a small airplane into the building where he worked – an IRS office in Austin, Texas – killing himself and a fellow worker.[26] He left a suicide note online that ended with the words (in *Suicide Stack*, Claire Fontaine project this note onto a screen so that it looks like the closing credits of a film):

I saw it written once that the definition of insanity is repeating the same process over and over and expecting the outcome to suddenly be different. I am finally ready to stop this insanity. Well, Mr Big Brother IRS man, let's try something different; take my pound of flesh and sleep well.

The communist creed: From each according to his ability, to each according to his need.

The capitalist creed: From each according to his gullibility, to each according to his greed.

Stack seems well aware that people may consider him to be insane, but in his eyes it is capitalism and the US Government that live up to "the definition of insanity." He is not committing suicide, he is being killed or – in the logic of (Antonin Artaud's book on) van Gogh – suicided by society. According to (t)his logic, Stack's suicide is not an indication but an interruption of insanity. Despicable as this may be, not least due to the fact that innocent people were hurt and killed, it is clear that Claire Fontaine finds the suicide letter interesting, and to a certain extent agrees with Stack's stark, very real, and visceral critique of capitalism.[27] Maybe, as Claire Fontaine suggests on a poster (*Untitled (What is freedom?)*, 2012), it is the capitalistic economy that could be said to be sick: "Why is capitalistic libidinal economy not a form of mental illness?"

Scene 2. The spectral temporality of capital

Frankfurt, autumn 2014: The exhibition *Unendlicher Spaß* (*Infinite Jest*) at the Schirn Kunsthalle. Referring to David Foster Wallace's novel *Infinite Jest*, the curatorial idea is to scrutinize the relation between, on the one hand, entertainment, enjoyment and euphoria, and on the other, despair, sadness and depression.[28] The background for the exhibition appears to be a society in which fun and happiness have developed into an ever-more intense imperative that tends to collapse into a state of exhaustion; just think of advertising slogans like Coca Cola's *Enjoy*, Nike's *Just do it* and Amazon's *Work hard, have fun and make history*. The question is: What if you are unable to do *it*, what if you do not have the energy to work and have fun and make history 24/7?

In one of the rooms three works by Claire Fontaine are on display. One of them is called *Untitled (The Invisible Hand)* (2011), a ready-made of a Newton's cradle, specially produced by Lehman Brothers. The cradle is in vogue among businessmen, directors and executives (as it says somewhere online: *executive playground!*)[29] Claire Fontaine has equipped this *objet trouvé* with batteries to maintain the constant pendulum movement of the small metal balls. Moreover, they have changed the base of the cradle so that it resembles a miniature tennis court, with white lines, a golden net and the word "networking" written humorously on the side. Above all this work is about movement and time in the finance economy.

The invisible hand, or the kinetics of capitalism
Back and forth they go, the silvery balls in Claire Fontaine's *Untitled (The Invisible Hand)*. Although it is actually only the two outermost balls that move. The three in the center are virtually still, while one of the other two swings to the side, only to

come back and hit the three in the middle, setting the fifth in motion. It is like a tennis match: The spectators turn their heads to one side of the court, then to the other, then back again. This pendulum movement is, however, more than an allusion to the (upper class) game of tennis. It could, evidently, also be said to resemble the perpetuum mobile of contemporary capitalism. The steady, endless, accumulative movement of capital. Everything is a means to a means, movement for the sake of movement, production for the sake of production, consumption for the sake of consumption, circulation for the sake of circulation. Marx already wrote in *Capital* that money performs the function "of a *perpetuum mobile* of circulation," and that "the circulation of money as capital is [...] an end in itself, for the expansion of value takes place only within this constantly renewed movement. The circulation of capital has therefore no limits."[30] In a similar vein, Moishe Postone argues that "[p]roduction in capitalism becomes a means to a means [...] The goal of production in capitalism is an absolute given that, paradoxically, is only a means – but one that has no end other than itself."[31]

This is the secret kinetics of the capitalist system shown by Claire Fontaine in *Untitled (The Invisible Hand):* To keep the system in motion no matter what (thereby ensuring endless accumulation). As with the gamblers in Vegas in the preceding chapter, one only plays to keep playing. That is all there is to the addictive, compulsive, almost pathological rhythm of capitalism – the only difference being that gamblers usually go home broke, while good capitalists get rich. Inevitably, though, this kind of kinetics betrays a certain stasis at the heart of the matter. The pendulum of the cradle in actuality makes manifest an infinite movement on the spot: It literally goes nowhere at all. Everything changes, and yet everything stays the same. All that moves remains in place.

In my reading, *Untitled (The Invisible Hand)* shows how capitalism today operates not only at the level of things but at the level of time itself. In recent years, a wide range of thinkers have made analyses of the contemporary regime of debt that support and supplement the one made by Lazzarato in relation to the temporal changes resulting from that regime. Although approaching the problem from a different angle, this is what Bernard Stiegler is preoccupied with in several of his books, most notably in *For a New Critique of Political Economy* in which he conceives of credit as the ultimate form of economic protention. According to Stiegler, the debt and speculation that permeate not only the financial economy, but the economy and society as a whole, annihilate the future if one perceives and conceives of the future as something *indeterminate*. "As pure calculation, it denies the very possibility of a future, given that the future cannot be calculated because it is essentially indeterminate: a calculable future is no longer a future but just the consequence of the present."[32] Taking an analogous approach, Joseph Vogl argues in *The Specter of Capital* that the algorithmic models driving financial speculation – futures, derivatives etc. – are a way of "taming time" and in particular the future, which is even more visible and violent when it comes to debt. In that sense, the title indicates that the ghost of capital is not a ghost from the past but from the future. As Vogl states in an interview, in an inversion of the famous opening lines of the communist manifesto (an inversion that he picks up from Don DeLillo's 2003 novel *Cosmopolis*): "It is a future of mounting debt that comes to weigh on the present. The 'spectre of capital' does not come out of the past, but rather as a memento out of the future and back into the present."[33]

But the spectrality or hauntology of *Untitled (The Invisible Hand)* works in a slightly different way. Here, the mechanical necessity that Newton ascribed to the natural laws seems to have been transferred to the economy. In "On some of the affects of capitalism," which I commented on in the chapter on Houellebecq, Bruno Latour maps out precisely the way in which the traditional relationship between nature – "binding necessities" – and capitalism – "boundless possibilities" – has today been turned upside down. In the words of Latour, economy and Earth have switched roles for good: "It is the Earth that is undergoing subversion at a dizzying pace and the Economy – that is, second nature – that still runs like clockwork."[34] Especially notable is the fact that, even after the bank crises and crash of 2008 of which Lehman Brothers more than any other came to be an emblematic symbol, the economy still runs like clockwork. This is the proper hauntological effect of Claire Fontaine's work: The cradle carries out and delineates a "ghost movement, that can now reproduce itself without human intervention, is a disquieting message that reaches us from an economic moment that has now past [sic] but that is still secretly alive and active under the skin of our present."[35] It is indeed a perverted version of the invisible hand, a zombiefied rendition of the Duracell Bunny, a capitalist automaton. It is magic!

No present(s)

What is at stake in *Untitled (The Invisible Hand)* is not only the pure abstraction of money, or the ever-more religious, if not magical character of capitalism, but the ways in which this development in the economic domain toward a system fueled by debt and financial speculation profoundly effects temporality as such.

This is also the reason that so many of Claire Fontaine's works deal explicitly with temporal questions, which is just another way of saying political questions. In neon works such as *Past Present Future* and *Please God Make Tomorrow Better,* Claire Fontaine hints at a global and contemporary situation in which the combination of debt and financial speculation seems to make the future a calculable and profitable domain for a small elite, and a source of endless desperation and depression for the rest.[36] At the 4th Thessaloniki Biennale of Contemporary Art, Claire

Fontaine's *P.I.G.S* was accompanied by a neon work of theirs that read "No Present." Obviously re-appropriating the "No Future" catchphrase of the punk movement, the work by Claire Fontaine, in the astute words of the curators:

> refers to the economical and historical conjuncture that sees many countries and their inhabitants deprived not only of a future but also of the possibility of a daily life that isn't just survival. The debt caused by the greed of a few in fact burdens entire populations, obliterating the minimal rights for millions of people, such as getting married, leaving one's parents' house or hoping to get a job. It can legitimately be said that now there is no present in a similar sense that the Sex Pistols used to sing "No Future." The present is always something shared and collectively created; a sum of solitudes only creates an absence of the present, the impossibility of its narration and the difficulty to grasp its transient consistency. No Present also has a double meaning, which is "There are no presents for anyone," as this is a time where everything must be earned and often at an unfair price.[37]

In the chapter on David Foster Wallace there was also talk of debt and of a present, in both senses of the word, but here the terms acquire a rather different meaning. A Kierkegaardian idea of infinite debt as an antidote of love to the pathology of depression would, in the eyes of Claire Fontaine, be absolutely meaningless in the current situation and, what is worse, inevitably lead to a voiding of the political as such. A generalized condition of debt precisely carries with it, to quote Lazzarato, a preemption of the future, a reduction of "what will be to what is."[38] According to Claire Fontaine, though, it seems that our present misery is not due to the fact that we have lost the future, but rather the present. Significantly, the sign does not read "No Future" but "No Present." So what if the problem is not that what will be is reduced to what is (in the sense that the future is nothing but a continuation and confirmation of the present) but that what is is reduced to what will be (in the sense that the speculative projections of financial capitalism eradicate the present as such by over-determining it in a kind of spectral feedback loop)? Then what needs to be done something about is the present.

To be sure, the small ready-made *Untitled (The Invisible Hand)* is not exactly an optimistic piece of art. The question of what *is* to be done must be followed by a question of what *can* be done. And the answer that Claire Fontaine provides in this work – and, more or less, in their practice as a whole – is: Not much. Though the work is cleansed of any subjective feelings and affects, there is a certain affectivity at play in the work: An affect of hopelessness, or impotence, which is less subjective than structural, implying among other things that it is not easy to say whether the impotence must be ascribed to financial players, avant-garde artists or the workers of the world. What is certain is that *Untitled (The Invisible Hand),* as already mentioned, functions as a critical comment on the eerie clockwork of capitalism but the work seems to be conscious of the impotence of this criticism at the same time. The work thus comes to reflect the fiscal and financial crisis exemplified by Lehman Brothers, as well as a crisis within art around its ability to really do anything about that crisis. In that sense, the empty, abstract movement of the balls occasions a depressed feeling that not only pertains to capital but to art itself: The sad little monotonous movements of the balls swinging back and forth are also somewhat telling and symptomatic for contemporary artists like Claire Fontaine, who find themselves incapable of doing anything about the capitalist clockwork, condemned as they are to participate in – and to a certain extent reproduce – a game that is totally rigged in the first place.

However, neither *Untitled (The Invisible Hand)* nor the other two works with which Claire Fontaine participated in the exhibition in Frankfurt addresses the problematic of depression directly. But numerous of their other works do exactly that. For example, *Study for pill spill (Prozac)*, an installation or sculpture of piles of anti-depressants (2010); *Vivre! Vaincre soi-meme, la depression (Brickbat)*, a brick wrapped in the cover of a French self-help book named simply *Vivre! Vaincre soi-meme, la depression* (which can be roughly translated as "Live! Defeat depression yourself") and, believe it or not, written by a person named Claire Fontaine (2006); and *Untitled (Why your psychology sucks)* (2015), a pungent and quite comical criticism of the self-help industry's ideological personalization of depression and generalized responsibilization of the subject.

Scene 3. Why your psychology sucks

Why are you depressed? What is the cause of your depression? What is the root cause? And what are some of the ways that you can start to get a handle on it? Depression is an epidemic. It's out there. So many of us, especially in first world countries nowadays, are starting to actually get more and more signs of depression.

Why is this going on? What's happening here? What's the rock bottom truth about depression? All right, here's the deal. I wanna be blunt with you here, 'cause the bottom line is, the reason you're depressed is because your psychology sucks. All right? You've got shit psychology. Now, I'm not blaming you, I'm just telling you a fact [...] you're causing your own depression.[39]

This is a transcription of a monologue from the beginning of the video work *Untitled (Why your psychology sucks)* by Claire Fontaine. The person speaking in the video is an African-American woman wearing a black suit and a white shirt. She is not an authentic self-help authority, though she certainly sounds like one. She is an actress, performing or reciting a text lifted word for word from a presentation by a man called Leo Gura – I suppose the surname guru would be a bit too much – who is, according to his Twitter profile, "a professional self-development junkie, life coach, video blogger, entrepreneur, and speaker." Gura, a bald man with a beard and founder of actualized. org, where the video *Why Am I Depressed?* and accompanying transcript can be found, helps "people design awesome lives" (again taken from his Twitter account). This is the source of the performance in the ready-made video, lasting a little more than 20 minutes, the critical point of which is how it entails a specific form of subjectivation that seems to correspond perfectly to the neoliberal economy.

"You are causing your own depression"

In the video by Claire Fontaine, the female actor acts with great determination and persuasive power, gesturing like a person who is trained to speak and trained to sell. That her message is quite strong should surprise no one, given that the subtitle of the original video by Leo Gura is "The Shocking Truth About Depression." The core truth of her message is that if one is depressed there is only one person to blame: "You are causing your own depression," the woman boldly declares. There is something wrong with your mental and cognitive apparatus, your psychology is "shit." Stop being a victim and take ownership of your psychology, she exclaims at one point. The logic of her speech is simple: People create their own reality. Thoughts alone can change things (not unlike the mind-cure movement that William James spoke about earlier). This means that *you* weave the thread of your own fate, there are no external circumstances and no excuses either.

What is the solution then? It ought to be mentioned that, at the beginning of the video, the speaker, having said that depression is an epidemic, makes a somewhat careful distinction between clinical cases of depression involving biological and genetic factors and "the other half of people," the overwhelming majority of the depressed, who are really just in a "bad psychological state." It is the latter group of people she addresses in the video. The solution for them is not psychiatry or psycho-pharmaceuticals but simple meditation. The solution is to be (in the) present. Here is what she has to say:

Take this exercise for example: If right now you dropped your past history completely, I mean forget about it, at least for a second, forget your past history, forget your future history, forget that you have a future, forget you have a past. Be completely in the moment right now. Get rid of every single thought that you have in your mind. Get rid of your idea of yourself. Pretend like you are dead. You have no more life. You have no more ego. You have no more conceptualizations. You have no more beliefs about how the world is, and how it works. And you just sit in peace and quiet.

In the video *Untitled (Why your psychology sucks)*, the viewer, the you of the video, is the *cause* of his or her own depression, but consequently also the only *cure*.[40] The point of meditating is to get rid of the ego, to get rid of yourself by pretending "like you are dead." There is "a lot of deep stuff here," she admits once more, and it is definitely not going to be easy, but it is worth it. These daily exercises can, in the long run, not only help you overcome depression but help you, more generally, to "master your psychology" and eventually put you in a state of "total bliss and happiness." It is a deeply moral message. Failing to be happy is simply immoral (a similar logic is at work in von Trier's *Melancholia*).

As a ready-made or re-enactment *Untitled (Why your psychology sucks)* is a pungent and quite comical criticism of the self-help industry's ideological personalization of depression and generalized responsibilization of the subject as such. These two tendencies cannot be stressed too strongly: Personalization and responsibilization. They go hand in hand. In his text, "Good for Nothing" from 2014, Mark Fisher, who was very attuned to this logic, or should I say tactic, wrote that depressed people are encouraged to feel and believe that their depression is their fault and their fault alone: "Individuals will blame themselves rather than social structures, which in any case they have been induced into believing do not really exist" – implicitly referencing Thatcher's claim that society does not exist.[41] This is precisely where the problem of depression feeds into a more general problem: The model of subjectivity advocated in the original self-help video by Leo Gura is identical to the model of the autonomous, self-determining, competitive individual, the fiction of capitalist, neoliberal subjectivity. The model of an indebted subjectivity, which makes the subject infinitely responsible for his or her own future. The indebted subject, as someone who makes a promise, becomes "answerable for his own *future!*" as Nietzsche emphatically formulated it in the lines from *On the Genealogy of Morality* quoted above.[42]

An ideological interpellation thus takes place in the video, which interpellates the subject as a subject and not as an object. As The Invisible Committee writes in their book *To Our Friends:* "We shouldn't think they are out to *destroy* us. We should start rather from the hypothesis that they're out to *produce* us."[43] This expands on a thought already present(ed) in the book *The Coming Insurrection* where they argue that in a society "where production no longer has an object," everything becomes a question of "[p]roducing oneself," because "[i]deally, you are yourself a little business, your own boss, your own product."[44] This is indeed the view that the female in the video promotes. You are your own boss, even when it comes to mental illness.

Moving beyond the stalemate of critique
(get rid of your self)

It is one of the clear aims of the ready-made video by Claire Fontaine not to criticize this kind of grotesque self-help discourse from without, but rather to let that discourse speak for itself, thereby exposing its defects and self-contradictory logic to the point where it becomes grotesque and rather comical. If one consults the original presentation by Leo Gura, it gets worse (or better). Here, after a short introduction, a flashing sequence of catchphrases or keywords momentarily interrupts Gura's speech. In the order given the words read: "Success, happiness, self actualization, life purpose, motivation, productivity, peak performance, creative expression, financial independence, emotional intelligence, positive psychology, consciousness, peak performance, personal power, wisdom." (Apparently, the concept of a "peak performance" is so important that it must be repeated).

Criticism of this particular discourse, so dominant in the Western world of today, admittedly feels a little cheap and ultimately rather unsatisfying, as Claire Fontaine herself seems all too aware. One of their other works, *Untitled (Stalemate)*, is a chessboard placed vertically on a wall with the remaining pieces caught in a situation of stalemate, a dead end of the game where neither white nor black can win, the analogy being that this critical disclosure of the self-help ideology can all too easily end in aesthetic, as well as political stalemate. That is not to say, however, that Claire Fontaine relinquishes a critical stance as such. Contrary to many contemporary artists and critics who seem all too satisfied to abandon a critique altogether, with reference to its anachronistic, suspicious, paranoid and rigid character, Claire Fontaine wants to hold on to the political potential of art regardless of how impossible that might seem today. In a way, this is precisely the impossible position in which Claire Fontaine has placed herself in her attempt to escape the stalemate, or what Ben Davis has called the Manichaeism of contemporary art in his book *9.5 thesis on art and class*: "The Manichean position of seeing art as either commercial and corrupt or noncommercial and pure."[45] In an interview Claire Fontaine – always able to conduct analytical and theoretical conversations about their own art – state the problem and their solution to it as follows:

> Our strategy consists in refusing to go and die in the countryside, refusing to believe that intellectual and aesthetic space are the private property of the entertainment industry, refusing to believe that a radical-political position can only exist on the level of direct action and its tragic consequences, and that the rest is an opportunist and pathetic gesticulation

[...] For radical people our attitude is a compromise, for conservatives it is a fraud, this logic must be exploded: it is literally bringing people to suicide.[46]

There is thus no question of Claire Fontaine wanting to initiate or realize an immediate passage to direct action; as well as rejecting the idea of a withdrawal into a politically passive position *within* the aesthetic domain, they refuse the opposite idea of an exit *from* art in favor of a purely political practice.

Going back to *Why your psychology sucks*, it should be clear by now how the female speaker's *personalization* of depression stands in stark contrast to Claire Fontaine's *politicization* of depression. At the same time, though, it is strange to see how some of the themes at the end of the promotional video resonate with some elements of Claire Fontaine's own diagnosis and prognosis. "Who wants to just come out of a depression to a normal kind of life?" the female speaker asks, adding: "That's probably why you were depressed in the first place." One can easily imagine the artist duo subscribing to a statement like that (even if the very next sentences are: "You don't really have a strong sense of purpose. I want you to set some huge goals for yourself. I want you to set an amazing vision for yourself.") Similarly, some of the thoughts that appear in the passage on meditation are also present in other areas of Claire Fontaine's *oeuvre*, not least the idea that the cure to depression is to get rid of yourself and your self. "Get rid of your idea of yourself. Pretend like you are dead," as it is put in the video. *Get Rid of Yourself* is, incidentally, the name of a film made, not by Claire Fontaine, but by Bernadette Corporation, an artist collective that works in the same tradition as Claire Fontaine and also functions as the space where Claire Fontaine's works are shown in New York. Taking its point of departure in the so-called Black Bloc of the anti-globalization events in Genoa, Italy, during the G8 summit in 2001, *Get Rid of Yourself* is a kind of (anti-)documentary in a montage form: Image and text, voice-over and dialog, actors and "real" protesters are incorporated within a zone of indistinction so radical that there is no way of discerning who is saying what. At the beginning some sentences run across the screen: "They say, 'another world is possible.' But I am another world. Am I possible?" At another moment a voice says (in French): "You're no longer a subject, the points of reference are lost." This is the point of the film: To be rid of all reference, all identity, and all sense of self-hood. Later, a female voice says (in English) that this process is all about "de-sub-jec-tiv-i-zation":

> to become opaque, extracting ways of living and of fighting so that, at a chosen moment, I test this slight displacement. I become a-whatever-singularity. Everything that isolates me as subject, as a body endowed with a public configuration of attributes, I feel it dissolve, bodies fray at their edges, at their limit they blur. Little by little, I achieve a new nakedness. That's what our need for communism is. A need for nocturnal spaces, where we can find each other beyond our qualities.[47]

The references here – and clearly Bernadette Corporation have not abandoned intertextual references – are not only to Agamben's concept of the whatever-singularity, but also to Robert Musil's *The Man without Qualities* and Herman Melville's Bartleby who would prefer not to. What is interesting about the Black Bloc, according to the movie itself, is that "everybody is looking the same so it is far more difficult to spot out...uh... individuals", as an English voice-over tells the viewers in an exaggerated stutter. According to this logic, the sentence "pretend like you are dead" must instead be read; pretend like your self is dead. To be without qualities, to get rid of yourself, is the ultimate political dream. Depression thus offers an opportunity in that it is a kind of "nocturnal space" in which subjectivity as such is dissolved. As The Invisible Committee puts it in their usual bombastic fashion: "We are not depressed; we're on strike. For those who refuse to manage themselves, 'depression' is not a state but a passage, a bowing out, a sidestep towards a *political disaffiliation*."[48]

This is where the concept and practice of the *strike* enters the picture. Is depression a form of strike and if so how? Is art to be considered work or rather refusal of work? What is the relation between art, depression and the political economy?

Scene 4. The human strike

"Grève humaine" is the French expression for "human strike," designating the most generic movement of revolt against any oppressive condition. It's a more radical and less specific strike than a general strike or a wildcat strike.

Human strike attacks the economic, affective, sexual and emotional positions within which subjects are imprisoned. It provides an answer to the question "how do we become something other than what we are?" It isn't a social movement although within the uprising and agitations it can find a fertile ground upon which to develop and grow, sometimes even against these.

For example, it has been said that the feminist movement in Italy during the 1970s demolished the leftist political organisations, but what hasn't been said is what leftist political organisations were doing to the women who were part of them. Human strike can be a revolt within a revolt, an unarticulated refusal, an excess of work or the total refusal of any labor, depending on the situation. There is no orthodoxy for it. If strikes are made in order to improve specific aspects of the workers' conditions, they are always a means to an end. But human strike is a pure means, a way to create an immediate present here where there is nothing but waiting, projecting, expecting, hoping.[49]

The practice of Claire Fontaine can be divided into several dimensions and domains; or perhaps it would be more accurate to say that their practice encompasses dimensions and domains that are normally separated in capitalism's infinite parceling out of specialized working tasks. Thus, the production of theoretical texts is an integral and essential part of their operation, which is why this scene is an essay, included in order to stress the fact that in the case of Claire Fontaine, it is no longer possible to uphold a traditional distinction between (art) theory and (art) practice, or between art and literature for that matter. The text in question, "Human strike has already begun," features in the book *Human Strike Has Already Begun & Other Writings* (2013) and is part of an ongoing meditation on what Claire Fontaine conceptualizes as *a human strike*.

The pure means of the human strike

Scholars generally agree that the "classical" strike crystallizes the fundamental conflict of the industrial age in the sense that it is the manifestation of where "the abrupt Marxian clash of capitalist class and proletariat was most neatly imaged."[50] Admirable as that form of strike was and is, it is on the verge of becoming an empirical impossibility, given the almost vegetative state of unions today, for example.[51] However, the pivotal point is that even if the unions still enjoyed the strength and support they used to, the strike would not be an adequate response to the current state of affairs according to Claire Fontaine. In contrast to the traditional strike form, the human strike is not a strike "reserved to" the proletariat, nor does it "merely" deal with, and protest against, working conditions and the modes of capitalist production: "Its subject isn't the proletarian or the factory worker but the whatever singularity that everyone is."[52] For Claire Fontaine, the human strike is not confined to the factory or to one's working life. It bears upon life as such; life as a whole. It is characterized by *totality*. Why this total character? Because of the generalization of a situation in which it is impossible to distinguish between work and life, and between work on the self and simply work. Because the economy of debt casts people as human capital and entrepreneurs, and saturates life in its – libidinal – entirety. Because man – if there ever was such a thing as man without quotation marks – under these current conditions, is no longer tormented by cold capitalism, alienation in and of the factory, or the estrangement from the product of his or her work, but a warmer and more emotional form of exploitation, where the reality is that "man" is too close rather than too distanced from his or her work; that is to say, his or her life.

Or so goes Claire Fontaine's analysis. In short: The human strike is an act of rebellion as the strike always has been, but the context for the human strike is a neoliberal economy in which subjectivity as such is at stake. In Claire Fontaine's own words, the human strike thus "attacks the economic, affective, sexual and emotional positions within which subjects are imprisoned."[53] In this sense, the human strike assumes a fundamentally affective quality. At the same time, it recoils upon a certain self-destructivity and acknowledges that the people who go on strike are by definition inscribed and entangled within society, a strike against which would imply that this strike must also necessarily be turned inwards against the striking subject itself. The human strike so to speak has to assure that it destroys those parts of the striking subjects that are nothing but the embodiments of a surrounding society, which was and is the target of the strike in the first place. Thus, the striking subject is both the subject and the object of the strike; the critical gesture of the strike demands a dose of self-criticism or – one of Claire Fontaine's key concepts – a process of *desubjectivation*, a process through which the striking subject gets rid of him or her self. As a direct consequence, the human strike can never be "an affirmation of the individual against the system," as one half of Claire Fontaine, Fulvia Carnevale, expresses it in a conversation with the artist John Kelsey, who is acutally part of the Bernadette Corporation.[54]

This is the condition for the human strike. It involves the whole of life and not just work. Better yet, it concerns work, insofar as work has invaded and become identical with the whole of life. Furthermore, the human strike is distinguishable from previous forms such as the general strike and the wild cat strike, by not having any particular *goal,* which not only makes it less specific, but also more radical. This means, firstly, that the strike is to be considered an instance of what Giorgio Agamben calls pure means, means without ends, and secondly, that the strike is not oriented toward the future, only toward the present. As Claire Fontaine herself writes: "The reflex of refusing any present that doesn't come with the guarantee of a reassuring future is the very mechanism of the slavery we are caught in and that we must break. To produce the present is not to produce the future."[55]

This should give one reason to pause for a moment, because it might come across as a bit odd. If the analysis is that we live in a world in which debt and financial speculation have confiscated the future and occupied every inch of the – individual and collective – imagination, would that not necessitate an emancipatory politics which had as one of its primary aims an opening toward other horizons, alternative futures? But as witnessed earlier, this is not quite Claire Fontaine's analysis. Although Claire Fontaine's diagnosis of the times may seem to dwell upon a loss of the future, their main concern is actually a loss of the present. In their eyes, the problem today is that there is No Present, rather than No Future. In fact, the slogans "human strike" and "sell your debt" could, and indeed should, be seen as attempts to refuse to participate in any (re)production of the future as such. Why help neoliberal capitalism with restoring a future that would merely end up as more of the same? That accounts for the temporality of the strike, which involves a suspension of any kind of progressive or teleological notion of time. The strike thus possesses a certain rhythmic quality; a rhythm of interruption. It becomes a temporal hole in itself, a negative eternity, a crisis in and of time, nothing but pure *durée,* approximating in the last resort – if not to begin with – a rejection of the (fantasy of the) future. This is where depression and strike become one. As a dissolution of the (identity of) self, including its temporal coherence, depression can and indeed must be seen as an exemplary strike form. Depression, in Claire Fontaine's work, is in and of itself a process of desubjectivation.

Work and art (Stop making art!)

But what about art? What is the relation between the art work and the human strike? Is art work? Is the artist a worker? And if so, what class does she belong to? Is she working class, part of the contemporary precariat as some suggest, or is she rather, as Ben Davis argues, "the representative of middle-class creative labor par excellence."[56] Of course, many artists have jobs on the side that could be said to be working class, but the artistic work in itself is, according to Davis, middle class: "This kind of intimate connection with the products of one's labor is exactly what working class people are denied by definition as a result of the quid pro quo that forms the central dynamic of a capitalist economy: trading your labor power for a wage."[57]

However, perhaps such questions are not particularly relevant in this context, for would it not be possible to understand art as refusal of work by its very nature; a superfluous activity or a radical inactivity? A supreme strike? Only if one completely disregards the commodity-based economy of which contemporary art is inherently part. In any event, it seems clear that the artistic strike, the refusal to work, actually requires a great deal of work. Unless, of course, the artist in question literally and *de facto* stops working, and ceases to produce art at all. This was what German artist Gustave Metzger tried to do in 1974 when he encouraged fellow artists to support an Art Strike that was to last no less than 3 years, from 1977 to 1980. These years without art were to be based on the premise that the artists who had accepted the challenge would no longer make or sell art, or participate in exhibitions, and thus no longer *be* artists, except perhaps an artist that had abandoned art: Paradoxically, the ultimate indication of a true artist. It is safe to say that Metzger's project did not receive a broad support; ostensibly not a single artist joined him in his strike. Regardless, the strike that Claire Fontaine has in mind is altogether different. It is obviously possible to regard the ready-mades as some sort of strike, but that does not get to the heart of the matter. What Claire Fontaine proposes is more a strike in relation to (the production of) artistic subjectivity and identity. As they write in the text "Ready-Made Artists and Human Strike: A few Clarifications," the point of departure for their strike is not so much the production of objects – the artworks – as the production of subjects – the artists. In the tradition of Italian feminists from the 1970s, Claire Fontaine envisions "a strike that would be an interruption of the relations that identify us and subjugate us more than could any professional activity."[58] This is the kind of interruption initiated by the reconfiguration of the artist as a ready-made artist, or of the artist as an assistant, in the sense given to the word by Giorgio Agamben. The artists themselves must get rid of themselves; they must pass through a fundamental transformation, or more specifically, a fundamental reduction or self-destruction.

Allow me to move on by going a little astray: At the end of an essay on art and activism on *e-flux*, Boris Groys refers to Michel Foucault's lectures on the birth of biopolitics (1978-1979), which in reality were lectures on the birth of neoliberalism and the – at the time relatively new – concept of human capital as the utopian horizon for contemporary capitalism. The reason that Groys goes into those lectures is that he is interested in how different artists have responded to these ideas. His primary example is Joseph Beuys – another artist who was in his prime in the 1970s: "At the beginning of the 1970s, Joseph Beuys was inspired by the idea of human capital. In his famous Achberger Lectures that were published under the title Art=Capital (Kunst=Kapital), he argues that every economic activity should be understood as creative practice—so that everybody becomes an artist."[59] What Beuys wanted to do was to make "the expanded notion of art" coincide with "the expanded notion of economy," so that the boundary between the two collapsed and everybody became an artist. The historical irony of this remarkable – though in retrospect rather naïve – project is that it turned out to be merely grist to the mill of neoliberalism: There is nothing neoliberalism would prefer more than to see all workers transformed into artists and creative entrepreneurs. As Hito Steyerl writes in the essay "Art as Occupation: Claims for an Autonomy of Life": "To push the point: life has been occupied by art, because art's initial forays back into life and daily practice gradually turned into routine incursions, and then into constant occupation. Nowadays, the invasion of life by art is not the exception, but the rule."[60] Referring directly to Beuys's dream, Patricia Reed makes a similar argument: "If 'the artist' has become a paradigmatic figure of contemporary labor, with no separation between life and work, then Joseph Beuys's clairvoyance has proven perversely accurate: we are all now indeed artists."[61]

What is central for Groys in "O Art Activism" is that contemporary conditions have changed to such a degree that the task of art today can no longer consist of a potentialization of human creativity, or in trying to make things or people *better*. Nor is an avant-gardistic unification of art and life to be desired. On the contrary, artists today must realize that their task is to make things worse. As Groys adds, "not relatively worse but radically worse." For Groys, it is "this artistic, social, and political alpinism" demonstrated by Beuys, that due to the historical changes having taken place in the meantime, must now be laid aside. An art that wants to be politically relevant at the present time "does not develop 'human potential' but annuls it. It operates not by expansion but by reduction."[62]

Groys does not mention depression in his text, but from my perspective it is nearly impossible not to interpret his text in this direction. When for instance, he writes that art should not develop but annul human potential, and that art should operate by reduction rather than by expansion, he seems to be describing the kind of depressive art that Claire Fontaine carries out. As a contemporary strike form, or as an emblematic example of the human strike, depression in itself appears to involve and embody what Groys looks for: "A U-turn against the movement of progress, a U-turn against the pressure of upward mobility."[63] As pure immobility and inactivity, depression brings about a rhythmic suspension of the order of the world – a caesura, a desynchronization – which is not pathological but political in its temporal and affective consequences. As John Kelsey suggests in the aforementioned interview with Fulvia Carnevale: "Human strike can produce a sort of displacement that happens only by preferring not to be moved. In the heart of a movement or within a situation of enforced mobilization, the invention of a new immobility. Depression, too, can be a mode of human strike – a refusal to participate in the post-Fordist exploitation of our most human capacities."[64] Indeed, that is the refusal to work, the U-turn, the Bartleby-like inactivity, that Claire Fontaine seeks in depression. In "Ready-Made Artist and Human Strike: A few Clarifications" she thus writes: "Human strike proposes no brilliant solution to the problems produced by those who govern us if it is not Bartleby's maxim: I would prefer not to."[65] I would prefer not to work, not to get out of bed, prefer not to pay my debt...

The return of the depressed (Threshold)

Summing up, this chapter has been intently focused on how in certain works, Claire Fontaine depicts depression as a symptom of a society in crisis, and a symptom of a neoliberal economy that rests on the twin towers of debt and financial speculation. It is indeed possible to generalize debt beyond a strictly economic level. Debt entails a certain modulation of subjectivity and temporality – and a certain pathological structure too. Although there is a connection between the current state of affairs and the contemporary proliferation of the diagnoses of depression – not to mention the numbers of suicides in some countries in the Western world – my concern has not so much been empirical cases and epidemiological facts as it has been to dwell upon the way these interrelated problems are imagined and constructed at a cultural level in the particular case of the art of Claire Fontaine.[66]

As Lazzarato points out in *The Making of the Indebted Man*, highlighting the relation between temporality and subjectivity within the debt economy, "debt appropriates not only the present labor time of wage-earners and of the population in general, it also preempts non-chronological time, each person's future as well as the future of society as a whole. The principal explanation for the strange sensation of living in a society without time, without possibility, without foreseeable rupture, is debt."[67] In Claire Fontaine's work that "strange sensation" is akin to individual *and* collective depression.

Yet the phenomenon of depression in their work is not merely a symptom, a passive reaction or even a pathology of futurity that must be therapeutically cured. Claire Fontaine has deliberately renounced any strategy that involves a reparation or creation of the future, which marks a decisive shift with regards to the historical avant-garde. The relation to the future is not something to be repaired or (re)created in the world of Claire Fontaine; the symptom is not something to be erased so that the social, economic, political structure can afterwards keep reproducing itself, thereby probably prompting the same or a new symptom in due time. These last conjectures have been an attempt to understand (Claire Fontaine's understanding of) depression as a contemporary form of strike; a human strike that can actually be said to constitute – or delineate the contours of – a political act, at least insofar as depression does not correspond to "the secret texture of values, lifestyles and desires hidden by the political economy," discussed by Claire Fontaine in the text "Human strike has already begun." This also means that the human strike of depression is to be understood as pure means, having abandoned any "guarantee of a reassuring future," insofar as the incessant futurizing and endless reproduction of financial capitalism are what must be dodged or, destroyed. It is thus not only the case that the depressed person has every reason to be depressed, nor merely that depression becomes a fully legitimate action;[68] it is also to be understood that, according to Claire Fontaine, depression is a political reaction to the society of the present; a "normal" response to an "abnormal" society. Depression is the epitomization of an exhausted *No, I can't* in a world characterized by an atmosphere of an emphatic *Yes, I can.*[69]

However, one might wonder whether Claire Fontaine individual depression can be endowed with the collective dimension that has been integral to strikes throughout most of modern history. Perhaps it is rather the very historical passage from resistance to pathology to which one would need to be more sensitive here; to the historical transition from strike *to* depression. Perhaps it is a sign of defeat rather than defiance that whereas people in the past used to strike collectively, today they become depressed individually (with the consequence that any critique of the system seems to collapse into a critique of the self). It remains an open question.

One thing is certain: The depressive art of Claire Fontaine poses a persistent paradox. They are deeply critical toward the institution of art, yet continue to present their works within the four walls of the white cube. Their art calls for political action, yet puts on display its own political impotence *as* art. They work the avant-garde tradition but find themselves in a world where the avant-garde – from a certain perspective and to a certain extent – is not a solution but part of the problem; where the dream of the avant-garde has turned into a nightmare that, to quote Marx, weighs on the brain of the living. They invoke a human strike, yet do so by means of signs and language alone: A neon sign that reads STRIKE. What is certain is that the ready-made artists Claire Fontaine continue to oscillate between the resistance of depression and the depression of resistance.

Chapter 4

Happiness and the end of the world as we know it: Lars von Trier's *Melancholia*

Introduction

No more happy endings! That was Lars von Trier's cheeky catchphrase for his movie *Melancholia* when it premiered at the Cannes Film Festival in 2011. At first glance, the ending of the film is far from happy: In a spectacular apocalyptic event that takes place in the final scene the – hitherto unknown – planet Melancholia collides with Earth, manifesting the end of the world as we know it, including the life of the two main protagonists, sisters Justine (played by Kirsten Dunst) and Claire (Charlotte Gainsbourg), as well as the latter's son, Leo. In this sense, the film is an act of uncorrupted cinematic killjoy. No more joy or happiness; only shattering disaster, sheer catastrophe. However, as the title of the film suggests, the film is not only about the end of the world, but also about depression, specifically Justine's depression.[1] Thus, the first part of the movie is called "Justine."

Melancholia opens with a wedding in a grandiose setting. Justine is getting married to Michael (Alexander Skarsgård). It is supposed to be the biggest and best day of Justine's life but it is not. Indeed, she is quite miserable, a fact that does not escape the other guests, especially Justine's brother-in-law, John (Kiefer Sutherland). In his eyes, the way Justine behaves and the fact that she is so obviously and obtrusively *not* happy, is totally unacceptable. During a significant scene, John delivers an imperative of happiness to Justine: "You better be goddamn happy." Throughout the film this demand is persistently placed before Justine: You ought to be happy; you have no right to be unhappy. What is strikingly clear, however, is that this demand cannot be met in any way whatsoever within the depressive horizon of, not only Justine, but also the film as a whole. "I smile and I smile and I smile," says Justine at one point in a tone that is both wicked and wry.

The first part of the film closes with the end of the wedding. The second part – covering roughly 5 days and nights – closes with the end of the world. Some time after the wedding, Justine, in a state of extreme depression, returns to the estate of John and Claire where the wedding took place so that they can take care of her. It is during this second part of the movie – entitled "Claire" – that the planet Melancholia enters the scene. Until this point, it is only Justine who, occasionally gazing up at the sky, notices a strange new phenomenon, which the hard-headed John, in all his scientific certainty, has identified as Antares in the constellation Scorpio. "I am amazed that you can see that!", he exclaims. At the end of the first part of the film, however, Justine looks up again, realizing, as a threatening omen, that "Antares is no longer there."

By the beginning of part two it has become common knowledge that the astronomical object is Melancholia, but whether the planet's trajectory entails a collision or merely a so-called fly-by is still unknown, at least to the people *in* the movie, with the possible exception of Justine. The viewers know all too well that this planetary dance, this ethereal ballet through empty space, will have a tragic outcome, since the movie's 8-minute prologue features a series of tableaus, not quite still images but ultra-slow motion "prophesies," accompanied by the overture from Wagner's *Tristan und Isolde*. Due to this cinematic structure of ellipse, the apocalypse at the end is a repetition – though not a totally exact one – meaning that the spectator knows how it will end before it even begins.

The relation between disaster and depression, then, gradually moves to the forefront in the film and this chapter. The questions are: Why has von Trier chosen to make a movie with two parts, a movie about depression *and* apocalypse, and not a movie about only one or the other? Does Jameson's prediction – that it is easier to imagine the end of the world than the end of capitalism – literally come true in *Melancholia*? And the final one: Is the movie an optimistic or a pessimistic one? My perhaps somewhat surprising intuition is that it is indeed optimistic. Whereas Houellebecq's response to the problem of depression was techno-ontological, Wallace's ethico-spiritual and Claire Fontaine's radically political, von Trier's is cosmological and eschatological. In the face of depression and disaster, his movie provides an impetus for what I would call an eschatological hope. Thus the end, so the argument and conclusion go, is a surprisingly happy one.

Scene 1. Party like there is no tomorrow

There is this one shot of Justine, sitting at her own wedding with an empty look in her eyes, while the guests dance and have fun. She is clearly not feeling well. She is depressed. But why is she depressed? Is it her off-putting job in the advertising business? Is it her husband, her family, her life, the world? In *Melancholia*, Lars von Trier refrains from offering any etiology, let alone any explanation. It is totally unclear why Justine suffers her depressive breakdown. But she does.

Some remarks on the tragedy and comedy of *Melancholia*

As a combination of Racine's Phaedra and Shakespeare's Ophelia, Justine seems to plod her way through the movie, the first part of which follows the wedding party of Justine and Michael as it proceeds, as the relations between the guests become increasingly awkward and a depression increasingly takes possession of Justine's body and mind. One of the images from the prologue that is not repeated in the remainder of the movie is of Justine lying in a river that carries her, ever so slowly, down toward the bottom of the screen in a perpendicular shot. She is wearing her wedding gown, eyes almost closed, the bridal bouquet still in her hands. Her veil billows in the water, where white water lilies also flow. The colors are green and white. Her predecessor is, of course, Ophelia from *Hamlet*. Like her, Justine is – in the words of Ophelia's mother, Gertrude – "incapable of her own distress," though unlike Ophelia, Justine's destiny is not a "muddy death." (act 4, scene 7). Nonetheless, the resemblance is striking and deliberate.[2]

The intertextual reference to Phaedra is far more implicit. But like Phaedra, it is as if Justine is carrying a weight that she cannot bear. Something is wrong with gravity, it seems; something is weighing her down. Like Phaedra, her legs tremble, she has trouble standing up, let alone walking. "These silly ornaments, these veils – the weight of them," Phaedra declares when we first meet her in Rancine's version of the story (1,3). Like Phaedra, Justine has the painful feeling that her clothes are too heavy, a burden to bear. In particular her wedding gown and bridal veil – those "silly ornaments" – appear to bother Justine throughout the evening, as epitomized by a shot from the prologue, in which Justine struggles to walk through one of the more overgrown areas of the estate. Some roots or lianas have wrapped themselves around her and intertwined with her bridal clothes until she is so entangled that it is nearly impossible for her to move at all, an impression reinforced by the very nature of the prologue with its ultra-slow images that occupy a space between photography and film. Justine later refers to this feeling, if not this image, in a conversation with her sister. She has just tucked her nephew into bed, and is so exhausted that she has decided to take a nap herself, when her sister enters the room, asking quite reasonably – it is Justine's wedding after all – what is going on. Justine replies in a flat almost dream-like voice: "I am trudging through this gray woolly yarn...it's...clinging to my legs. It is really heavy to drag along."

There is, in other words, a great deal of tragedy in *Melancholia*, though I want to be clear that I use the word tragedy in the completely ordinary sense of the word, not as a genre or a grandiose philosophical concept. As a character, Justine has a close kinship with tragic heroines such as Phaedra and Ophelia. All things do indeed "distress and hurt," as Phaedra complains at one point. At the same time, however, the movie has a certain comic quality, and this comedy is inseparable from Justine's depressive character, or perhaps more accurately, from the desynchronization between Justine and her surroundings; between her behavior and the expectations and conventions of the environment. It is a contrast that creates comedy. For example, when the wedding planner (played by Udo Kier, a long-time favorite actor of von Trier) cannot stand the sight of her because she ruins the party he has been hired to curate, and for that reason holds a hand before his eyes every time she is nearby. Or when the wedding cake cannot be cut because Justine is up in her room, taking a bath. Or when she cannot throw the wedding bouquet because she is, at this stage, in a state of catatonic depression, requiring her sister Claire to come to her aid, demonstratively hurling the bouquet from a balcony in her place.

According to Henri Bergson, comedy arises precisely when a human recalls a machine, when the animate approaches the inanimate, and when the human body appears as artificial and mechanical. The "deflection of life towards the mechanical," as Bergson writes in *Laughter*, is a "real cause of laughter."[3] Is this not exactly how Justine and her body appear in the first part of *Melancholia*? As an automaton, as something living a (non-) life of its own, alien to itself as well as to the people around it. In the movie, there is a comical gap between what one can and cannot do, physically *and* socially: What Justine wants to do is physically impossible; what she does do is socially inappropriate. In *Laughter*, Bergson quotes Napoleon's famous definition: "The transition from tragedy to comedy is effected by sitting down." This is the very transition that Justine carries out in the still above. In the midst of dancing guests, she has simply sat down to great comical effect. And yet there is something about *Melancholia* that is not funny at all, though, as Sianne Ngai and Lauren Berlant point out in the article "Comedy Has Issues," "the funny is always tripping over the not funny, sometimes appearing identical to it."[4] It is clearly not the direct variety of comedy of *The Kingdom* (*Riget*, 1994/1997), *The Idiots* (*Idioterne*, 2003), or *The Boss of it All* (*Direktøren for det hele*, 2006). The comedy of *Melancholia* is more flat and one-dimensional; indeed, at one point the laughter simply dies away, mutating into a fixed, mirthless smile.

Cinematic depression

Justine's psychopathological condition and the medium of film intersect in her slow physical movements (one hesitates to write the word in plural). Even the smallest movement is an Olympian struggle for her, and though psychomotor retardation is, of course, a well-known component of depression, in the case of Justine we have to take seriously the art form in which her depression appears. Cinema is, by its very definition, images in motion, and the prologue's ultra-slow images function not only as an indication of but as an intensification of Justine's depressive slowness.

It can safely be said that Justine incarnates a depressive temporality in the sense given to it by Thomas Fuchs, whose idea of a temporal desynchronization I have already refered to multiple times. His work still provides a helpful framework for understanding this desynchronization as "an uncoupling in the temporal relation of organism and environment, or of individual and society."[5] The most general characteristic of von Trier's aesthetic method in *Melancholia* is precisely a permanent juxtaposition of two temporal regimes. Almost every shot in the prologue is a juxtaposition, or perhaps more accurately, a superimposition of two images with two different temporalities, and thus two movements with different speeds. The background, for instance, is nearly completely still like a photograph, while something or someone in the foreground moves, albeit in the most minuscule and imperceptible way – or vice versa. Through this layering technique the prologue evidences a temporal disjunction; formally, the time is utterly out of joint. Two temporalities are constantly contrasted, from the human to the planetary level, where planet Earth and the planet Melancholia also belong to two discrete regimes of time (doublings saturate the entire movie: there are two planets, trees cast two shadows etc.).

One might specify the temporal desynchronization in *Melancholia* even further and say that everyone around Justine is engaged in one protentional activity or another, while she herself is not. They are all futurizing, planning ahead, drawing up possible scenarios. Her neurotic, uptight sister Claire organizes the course of events for the wedding; her brother-in-law, a severe caricature of an enlightenment man, tries meticulously to figure out astronomical trajectories and is all too willing to tell those around him about his latest conjectures; her boss, an incredibly unsympathetic ad man, wants Justine to come up with a tagline for a new advertisement; and so on. In the encounter with these characters and their respective futurologies, Justine emerges as fixated and observing. The world around her is in a perpetual transit between present and future, whereas Justine manages barely to withdraw to one of the estate's many rooms (Leo's bedroom, the bathroom etc.). However, this withdrawal occurs not only in the encounter with others' futurologies, but more precisely, in the encounter with the gaze of the others toward *her* future: Her mother, the perfect picture of a bitter divorcee, expects Justine's marriage to end in rapid and absolute failure – "Enjoy it while it lasts" – her sister announces the next item on her wedding-agenda – "We are going to move to the living room so that we can clear some tables. Then the newly-weds will dance, and, uh, then at 11:30 the bride and groom will cut the cake" – and her husband shows her a picture of a plot of land he has bought in Italy – "In ten years time, when the trees have grown, you can sit in the shade, in a chair, and if you still have days when you feel a little sad, I think that'll make you happy again…maybe we can have a little swing hanging from one of the trees."

On all of these occasions the camera pans very explicitly toward Justine's facial expression, which shows signs of an insurmountable obstacle. It is not that she does not *want* to meet the futurological propositions emanating from her family and friends; it is that she *cannot* understand and relate to them because, as a result of her depression, her very capacity for futurizing is absent. To imagine and plan *whichever* future is beyond her. Any appeal to this or that future is thus to be seen as a demand for the initiation of a speculative process, to which she – at the present point in time – does not have access. The depressed gaze – or at least Justine's gaze – does entail a gaze toward the future, but only in the sense of a gaze toward other people's gaze toward the future, and the request to participate in an act of speculation, with which such a gaze always seems to be concomitant. Justine is not only portrayed as a human being who does not have a future; she is a human being to whom depression *is* this loss of the future.

The tapestry of interwoven futures

It is now possible to summarize what is at stake in this first part of *Melancholia*. Because cinema is an art form that is distinguished by its engagement with time, depression in von Trier's movie is transposed into a negotiation between the temporality of the movie's images, the temporality of Justine and the temporality of the other characters. In this negotiation, Justine's experience of a frozen future is not only manifest as a purely psychological pathology; it is also asserted bodily, as a kind of slowness, inertness or pure immobility. The surrounding movements fixate her as immovable.

Justine's depression is characterized by a temporal desynchronization, a defect futurology, whose symptoms are rendered visible in the confrontation with an environment in which constant planning appears as a *sine qua non*. Through this mania of forward planning, often cast in a comical light, a certain model of subjectivity is drawn out according to which the subject is an animal who makes plans. In phenomenological terms, being is protentional. However, the many plans for the future that the characters frantically design are not strictly

163

speaking to be viewed as projections from a fixated temporal subject position, but rather as projections in a Heideggerrian sense, as *Entwurf*. To Heidegger being as such, *Dasein*, is a projection toward a futural field of possibilities. The notion of *Entwurf* is closely related to Heidegger's fundamental insight that being is ec-static, outside itself, besides itself, ahead of itself. This implies that any given human being is always coming from somewhere and going somewhere else, and that the present is thus blurred, flowing out into the future in advance in the form of expectations, hopes, projections and plans.[6]

In *Melancholia*, the people around Justine are, therefore, not so much subjects who make plans for the future; they make plans to the extent that they are subjects. But *Melancholia* differs from *Sein und Zeit* in at least one decisive way: The *Entwurf* in von Trier's movie is not a personal *Entwurf* alone, an already-in-the-future-being-with-myself. In Justine's interaction with the wedding guests it is evident that the futurology in question is necessarily a futurology addressed to others. In his book *Agonie des Eros,* in which the first chapter is devoted to an analysis of *Melancholia,* German philosopher Byung-Chul Han condenses this point into a single sentence: "Die Zukunft ist die *Zeit des Anderen* [the future is the time of the Other]."[7] But *Melancholia* is – unlike David Foster Wallace's work – not about the time of the *Other* or of the *other,* unless in a very abstract sense. The time of the *others* seems far more critical in *Melancholia*: (Planning for) the future is a social and collective affair. In fact, this forward planning holds social life together as such. When any given knot in the tapestry of interlaced and woven futures unravels, the whole thing falls apart, revealing, in that very moment, its *modus operandi.* This is what happens when Justine is no longer capable of sustaining the futurological network: The guests become angry, her husband leaves the wedding prematurely, and the whole social event is simply pulled to shreds.

One question remains, though: What is the purpose of this

never-ending planning? What animates all of the characters' plans, at least in the first part of the movie? The answer is simple: Happiness.

Scene 2. "I smile and I smile and I smile"

"I have never seen you look so happy," says Justine's father to his daughter at the beginning of *Melancholia*. Clearly, he does not know what he is talking about. It really takes a charlatan, whose charm as a human being is only equaled by his irresponsible and egoistic absence as a father, to fail to see that Justine is not happy at all. However, the truly remarkable feature of the movie, and Justine's depression, is not that her father is so full of himself that he fails to see what is right in front of him, nor that Justine is unhappy at her own wedding. Rather, what the movie wants to underline, it seems, is that Justine's depression is a thorn in the side of everyone else. It is as if her depression is a disruption to their planning fever; her unhappiness a violation of the moral imperative to be happy, above all and always.

"You better be goddamn happy"

"I smile and I smile and I smile," Justine desperately says at one point, having just been confronted by her sister, who wants an explanation: Why is she not happy, why is she constantly disappearing from the party (*her* party!), why can she not cut the wedding cake or throw her bridal bouquet from the balcony? Can she not at least pull herself together? But I try, Justine objects. She smiles and smiles and smiles. Her sister is not convinced one bit; in fact, this response infuriates her even more: You are lying to all of us, she exclaims.

If Claire – in all her patronizing passive-aggressiveness – is still the most understanding and gentle of all the people around Justine, this is only because the other guests are very explicit and even quite brutal in their reaction to Justine's demeanor. As mentioned, the wedding planner, for instance, cannot stand the sight of her, which he makes no effort to hide. But John, Justine's brother-in-law, is by far the worst. In a scene where Justine once again retreats to Leo's room, John is already there, sitting in the shadows as if waiting for her. It is here that he delivers the harsh line: "You better be goddamn happy." "Yes, I should be. I really should be," Justine – seemingly – complies. Still, John is not satisfied. The rest of the painful, cringeworthy dialog unfolds as follows:

> John: Do you have any idea how much this party cost me? A ballpark figure?
> Justine: No. I don't. Should I?
> John: Yes, I think you should. A great deal of money. A huge amount of money. In fact for most people, an arm and a leg.
> Justine: I hope you feel it's well spent.
> John: Well, that depends whether or not we have a deal.
> Justine: A deal?
> John: Yes, a deal. That you be happy.
> Justine: Yes, of course. Of course we have a deal.

In the end Justine is just too exhausted not to humor John. Yes, of course we have a deal, she says. Good, he says, kissing her on the cheek. Congratulations, he says and leaves her alone, whereupon Justine gives herself a fake smile in the mirror. Good girl.

Happiness as industry and ideology

In the danger of letting von Trier's movie hang in mid-air for a moment, some context must be provided. As Will Davies has shown in *The Happiness Industry* (2015), happiness has indeed developed into a real industry. Happiness, he writes, is what preoccupies our global elite.[8] National governments, as well as international business enterprises, are increasingly interested in the happiness – and health – of their populations and workers. Inspired by the work of positive psychologist Martin Seligman, David Cameron, for instance, while still prime minister of the

UK, wanted to create a national "happiness index." As he said when he launched the plan in 2010, "It's time we admitted that there's more to life than money and it's time we focused not just on GDP but on GWB – general well-being."[9] Although this may seem "woolly," as Cameron himself has admitted, with the re-union of economics and psychology in the early 1990s and advances within neuroscience, happiness is no longer to be seen as a fluffy, metaphysical concept, but rather a scientific concept that refers to a physical occurrence in the body, brain and behavior of human beings as such. Hence, what we are dealing with here is happiness in "an objective, measurable, administered sense."[10]

Of course, Cameron was not doing this purely for the sake of the British population; happiness, health and general well-being are a prerequisite for any effective capitalist production. The report *The Wellness Imperative – Creating More Effective Organizations* from the World Economic Forum, on the intimate connection between wellness and business, makes this abundantly clear: "Physical and psychological well-being is no longer treated as a free-floating desirable whose business benefits may (or may not) be realizable at some indeterminate point in time. Addressed at the level of structure, capacity and capabilities – of leadership and of people systems and processes – it becomes a powerful mechanism for translating strategy into measurable business performance."[11] Happiness – or in this context: "physical and psychological well-being" – is in other words not a peripheral priority, a by-product of a successful organizational structure, but something that must be addressed and dealt with on a *strategic and structural level*; something to be quantified, objectified and measured in order to deliver the best possible performance and ensure maximal profit. That happiness and health are a societal concern is beyond doubt; that depression and generalized unhappiness are an economic burden to society is also indisputable, despite the astronomical profits generated by the pharmaceutical industry worldwide.

Happiness, however, is more than an industry; it is an ideology, a moral imperative, a form of subjectivation. This is the reason Slovenian philosopher Alenka Zupančič develops the concept of "biomorality" in her book *The Odd One In,* where she nails the normativity of contemporary happiness: "A person who feels good (and is happy) is a good person; a person who feels bad is a bad person."[12] It should not be cause for surprise that multiple thinkers and writers have ventured into this particular problem. In *Smile or Die: How Positive Thinking Fooled America and the World,* journalist and activist Barbara Ehrenreich offers a critical yet entertaining account of the cult of positive psychology, optimism and happiness. Taking as a point of departure her experience of being diagnosed with breast cancer, and being surrounded by pink ribbons and an insistent demand to stay positive, Ehrenreich unfolds a wide range of psychological, cultural and economic implications that extend far beyond the domain of cancer patients: "If optimism is the key to material success, and if you can achieve an optimistic outlook through the discipline of positive thinking, then there is no excuse for failure. The flip side of positivity is thus a harsh insistence on personal responsibility."[13] In *The Wellness Syndrome,* Carl Cederström and André Spicer critically examine and provide ample humorous examples of how "happiness and health become the fundamental criteria for what passes as a moral life," and conceptualize this as an "insourcing of responsibility."[14] One element that each of these very different thinkers touches upon is the way in which positive psychology and the imperative of happiness entails a process of personal responsibilization, making each subject personally responsible for almost everything; success or failure, health or illness are a matter of subjective willpower, lifestyle and choice alone. As Claire Fontaine also made clear in their video *Untitled (Why your psychology sucks),* there is no "excuse for failure," as Ehrenreich points out. If you are such a bad person that you have become unhappy – or depressed – it is you, and you alone that is to blame.

Pascal Bruckner (Perpetual Euphoria: *On the Duty to Be Happy*) and Sara Ahmed (*The Promise of Happiness*) are two other authors who have also detailed how happiness has become one of the most dominant ideological imperatives today and how it is simply immoral to be unhappy. Now, "Life, Liberty and the pursuit of Happiness" is a well-known phrase from the United States Declaration of Independence. One might have good reason to object that life as such has the structure of a fantasy or a promise or that human beings "are the only beings for whom happiness is always at stake in their living, the only beings whose life is irremediably and painfully assigned to happiness," as Giorgio Agamben has suggested.[15] To return to Heidegger, one could even say that the notion of life as a promise is congruent with his idea that *Dasein* is, in the last instance, a constant projection (*Entwurf*), a perpetual anticipation (*Vorlaufen*), an anticipation of possibility, a leaning toward the future, or a running ahead of oneself.[16] That may very well be the case from an existential or ontological perspective, but the point here is that the futural promise of happiness upon life has changed character in recent years, and quite dramatically at that. No longer does the promise merely entail a possibility, however fantastical (as Heidegger, for one, would be the first to stress); rather, it is as if the promise of happiness has become an example of what Lauren Berlant would call cruel optimism. It is as if the very *possibility* of happiness has transformed over time into a social *necessity*, into a demand that in today's society is as economic as it is existential. In that sense, I am tempted to make an – admittedly ugly – synthesis of the two titles of Ahmed and Bruckner's respective books and consequently speak of a *promise* of happiness that has mutated into a *duty* of happiness.

The happiness contract

With this, the ground has been prepared for understanding why von Trier makes so much of the problem of happiness in *Melancholia*. It is beyond doubt that his movie deals seriously with happiness as some sort of biomoral imperative. This is the reason that the only character in the movie to have a relation to the outside world is an ad man, insofar as advertising is based upon what Berardi terms "imaginary models of happiness."[17] This is also the reason that all the characters are constantly planning their – near or distant – future: To sustain the fantasy of happiness, a fantasy that keeps their respective futurologies alive. Likewise, it is the reason that everyone asks, urges or even begs Justine to be happy. The people around her constitute a choir, persistently preaching a true gospel of happiness. However, John – a man who seems only to care about astronomy and money – really takes it to the next level. As noted above, he wants nothing less than to strike a deal with Justine, and to turn her happiness into a contractual obligation: He has paid a lot of money for the wedding – "an arm and a leg" – so he deserves that she "be happy." Her happiness is his right, and her duty. In this way happiness is transformed into a relation of debt: According to John, Justine simply owes him her happiness. A futural bind is thus created which is as economic as it is moral.

Of course, Justine cannot satisfy John's demand: She cannot keep to the contract and she cannot reimburse him with the currency of happiness. This is because the anticipation of possibility, so integral a part of life, is not available to her; her depressed being expresses absolutely no anticipation of possibility, no *"Vorlaufen in die Möglichkeit"* as Heidegger formulates it in the German original of *Being and Time*. She is not able to run ahead of herself; she is not able to run at all. Even walking and standing, as we have witnessed, is too much for her. For her, happiness is on another planet entirely.

Scene 3. Countdown, catastrophe

In *Thus Spoke Zarathustra*, Nietzsche wrote: "'We invented happiness' - say the last human beings, blinking."[18] But what do the last humans in *Melancholia* see when they stop blinking and open their eyes? They see a planet they have not seen before, a planetary dance of death that terrifies them. From that very moment - i.e. from the beginning of part two, "Claire" - it is all about the planet Melancholia. Will it pass by Earth in a so-called fly-by or will everything end with a cataclysmic collision? The countdown has begun. A more grandiose framework of futurology seems to have replaced that of all the petty plans for happiness that circulated in part one. Yet, as Heidegger knew, the radical horizon of *Dasein* is precisely death. But in the face of total annihilation, everyone is in it together. This means - *contra* Heidegger - that we are no longer dealing with the presentiment of *my own death* but with death of *us*, humanity as such, which makes the future (death) into a radically shared and collective matter. What, therefore, is the relation between the existential and eschatological, the phenomenological and the cosmological, the time of the soul and the time of the world, depression and disaster? How is the world going to end: With a whimper or a bang?

TINA

Why did Lars von Trier choose to make a movie about depression *and* the end of the world? A preliminary answer - in need of further elaboration - is that von Trier appears to depict depression as the personalized and pathological feeling that the future is closed off, frozen once and for all. "[T]he end of history will be a very sad time," Francis Fukuyama wrote laconically in his infamous essay "The End of History?" from 1989.[19] Yet Fukuyama had no idea of how sad it would really be. As both

Steven Shaviro and Mark B. Sandberg perceptively point out, von Trier's movie seems to index a contemporary situation in which history has ended and all that is left is the perpetual present of representative democracy and neoliberal capitalism.[20] There is no future, all there is is what is – "There Is No Alternative," as Margaret Thatcher triumphantly declared.

As noted earlier, this is what Mark Fisher conceptualizes as capitalist realism, i.e. "the widespread sense that not only is capitalism the only viable political and economic system, but also that it is now impossible even to imagine a coherent alternative to it."[21] Similarly, Franco "Bifo" Berardi has entertained a notion of depression as a symptom of "the present collapse of the imagination of the future," and Fredric Jameson has written extensively on a general "blockage of the historical imagination."[22] The problem, in other words, is not so much that nothing is left to the imagination, but that the imagination is left to nothing (*imagination dead imagine*, as Beckett once wrote). However, in von Trier's movie the absence of the future is not a conjecture, nor is it due to some imaginative deficit: It is pure fact. The humans in *Melancholia* literally have no future. The question posed by J. G. Ballard quite some time ago (in the *Daily Telegraph* in 1993) – "Does the future still have a future?" – is no longer a rhetorical question. Though the movie does not once mention climate change or global warming, it is impossible to ignore these contextual connotations when watching it. Clearly, the sense of living in a time with no future has only been reinforced in the age of global warming.[23] While global warming certainly feeds into the aforementioned problem of an atrophy of historicity – vividly conceptualized by Jameson as "the death of historicity" – it is important to take into account the specificity of the problem. As Sylvere Lotringer states in an interview: "The most disturbing aspect of our present situation is the disappearance of history —not the history of the past, but of the future. It is impossible for us to imagine that our history will have happened for no one."[24]

This is indeed the problem that *Melancholia* poses, notwithstanding its lack of explicit references to the current climate crisis. A history that will have happened for no one, but happened nevertheless. In grammatical terms, this fundamental condition is that of the future anterior: The inescapable fact that "there will *have been* humans," as Claire Colebrook writes.[25] This is the light in which human existence – the human species as a whole – is cast today. As Colebrook observes once more, we have obviously always known about our own mortality, and have always been aware that we are going to die some day, but now we have, in a certain sense, been given an expiration date. Here Colebrook refers to Mikhael Bakhtin, who apparently said, "the problem with the ancient Greeks was that they didn't know they were the ancient Greeks."[26] But we *know* that we are the last humans on Earth, give or take a few generations. Revisiting one final time Bruno Latour and his argument that nowadays "it is the Earth that is undergoing subversion at a dizzying pace and the Economy – that is, second nature – that still runs like clockwork," I want to paraphrase this and say that the Earth may not run like clockwork but the clock is ticking all the more so. This would be the reason why the last humans of today blink: They screw up their eyes and prefer to preoccupy themselves with being *happy* – for as long as it lasts – because they do not want to look reality in the eye. Alternatively, the last humans *roll their eyes* in a final act of post-modern irony. Either way, what they cannot endure is, not so much the brightness of the new day, as the utter darkness of the infinite night to come.

The Eschaton and the world-without-us (was Jameson right?)

Who could blame them though? Is it really so easy to look the end of the world in the eye? Going back to Jameson's famous statement that it has become easier to imagine the end of the world than the end of capitalism – a statement which has almost become a truism by now – I quite simply need to ask whether it still holds. An overwhelming number of *post*-apocalyptic movies would seem to indicate the opposite, and to confirm Jean Baudrillard's hypothesis – encountered in the chapter on Houellebecq – that the paradigmatic problem of our time is not that history has come to an end, but that history cannot end. All these cinematic depictions of worlds *after* the end of the world suggest that the end of the world was not *really* the end of the world after all.

In von Trier's *Melancholia* a constant struggle to establish the end of the world is played out. The prologue and the ellipse it creates is one such example. That we cannot take the end of the world for granted; that we perhaps need to revisit and reverse the established consensus that it is easier to imagine the end of the world than to imagine the end of capitalism, is further implied by the music of *Melancholia*. Steven Shaviro notes that "the music holds back from — or indefinitely postpones — the resolution and relief of a final cadence. The world is about to be annihilated; but when there is no prospect of a future, there is also no climax, no 'sense of an ending.'"[27] Instead of an instrumental piece of music building up to a concluding climax or crescendo, *Melancholia* is haunted by endless repetitions, and endless beginnings, as though the music itself is at a standstill, incapable of moving forward toward an end forever out of reach. It is not only in a visual or musical sense that von Trier plays with temporality, but also characterologically, in his choice of characters. As Sandberg has drawn attention to, the casting of Kiefer Sutherland in the role of John, and of the less well-known Brady Corbet as the advertising aspirant Tim – with whom Justine suddenly decides to have sex in the sand of the 19-hole golf course sometime during the wedding – is far from coincidental. Both appeared in the television series *24*, with Sutherland in the leading role as Jack Bauer. Sandberg suggests that this must be seen as a "radical play with the idea of incremental time" and as a "[t]ongue-in-cheek commentary on the idea of linear time and the countdown to catastrophe."[28] Thus, even though there is the sense of a countdown in the movie, of a clock ticking, of time running out, we should not forget this recurrent satirizing of the countdown scenario. Lars von Trier seems to take a slightly skeptical stance toward the inflation that has hit these virtual countdown dramaturgies. Throughout the film he plays with his characters' expectations and fears; at one moment the planet Melancholia seems to be moving away from the Earth, and the next it is approaching again. John actually constructs a gauge to be attached to the chest with which, after a 5-minute wait, one can see if the planet has moved closer or farther away. It is somewhat similar to the well-known, but essentially cruel, Freudian game, in which one repeatedly holds up a toy in front of a child, before hiding it behind one's back: Now you see it, now you don't: *Fort-da* on a planetary scale.

Yet, despite all the difficulties that the end of the world poses for the faculty of the imagination, and despite all the games on the part of the director, it all ends with a *bang*. The world ends, and so does the movie. It is an *Eschaton* quite different from that in Wallace's *Infinite Jest*, wherein it refers to a ridiculously complicated game played by students at the Enfield Tennis Academy. It would appear that what von Trier wants us as viewers to see, witness, imagine, understand, and fully and truly recognize, is indeed the end of everything. That it all ends here and that there is no possibility of any *post*-apocalyptic framework, since that would imply that things do continue, that there is a history after the end history, a time succeeding the end of time (in this sense, Shaviro is absolutely correct when he writes that *Melancholia* is a very *literal,* even *unironic* movie[29]). This is also where Houellebecq and Trier part ways, despite their shared preoccupation with the problem that Baudrillard, among others, has laid bare. In Houellebecq's writing we get a world that ends with a whimper, a slow death, a dream of immortality and a post-human after-life assisted by a radical ontological and technological change, and in terms of geography we get the landscape of *Possibility of an Island,* gently sloping for thousands of miles. Not so in von Trier's vision in *Melancholia*: Here we get the bang, the musical theme one final time, the planetary collision and then...Nothing. A black screen and no sound for approximately 10 seconds before the credits start to roll. Other than that, nothing; no after-life, no post-apocalypse. Nothing.

In his reading of this ending, Sandberg refers to Peter Szendy who has called *Melancholia* "the only rigorously apocalyptic film in the history of cinema,"[30] because the ending is so radical in its commitment to letting the last image really be the last image, and the last humans remain the last humans indeed. Shaviro takes a similar view, though he approaches the ending, and the film in general, from the perspective of what has become known as *speculative realism.* Drawing upon Ray Brassier's book *Nihil Unbound: Enlightenment and Extinction,* Shaviro argues that von Trier's movie confronts his viewers with "the literal truth of extinction."[31] As such, extinction lies beyond human experience, because we are no longer dealing with what can be conceived, experienced and thought by humans. There is literally no one left to experience and bear witness to the catastrophic event, which therefore, strictly speaking, cannot be called an event. It is simply irreducible to the correlation between world and man, object and subject. There are many synonyms within speculative realism for the spatio-temporal coordinates of extinction, which von Trier obviously cannot show but would nevertheless still seem to leave us with: The world-without-us, the thing-in-itself, the great outdoors, the omnipotence of chaos, an absolute outside, a purely glacial realm. In this analysis, the residual affect of *Melancholia* as a speculative movie is what Pascal, in his *Les* Pensées, called "the terror of the eternal silence of infinite space," a phrase of incitement, which Houellebecq by the way is also fond of quoting. One of the founding fathers of speculative realism, Quentin Meillassoux, deciphers Pascal's phrase as "the discovery that the world possesses a power of persistence and permanence that is completely unaffected by our existence or inexistence."[32] For Meillassoux (whom Brassier has translated into English), the primary concern is with the past, with a past before human existence – conceptualized as ancestrality – but in *Melancholia* the concern is with pure posteriority: A future with no human life; a future which persists indifferently, and regardless of the existence of humanity as such. This is what Shaviro intends when he writes that *Melancholia* "makes us aware of a universe that is not centered upon, or necessarily correlated with, humankind."[33] No (human) memorialization or conceptualization is available or adequate. It is in this sense that *Melancholia*, according to Shaviro, is a truly "'speculative realist' film."[34]

A nothingness to the nth degree?

It would appear to follow that von Trier's *Melancholia* is not only a speculative realist movie about the end of the world, but a deeply pessimistic, if not nihilist one. Inspired by the work of Eugene Thacker, Shaviro repeatedly refers to "von Trier's cosmic pessimism" and "von Trier's pessimistic aestheticism,"[35] which corroborates Sandberg's claim that "most critics read this total void as von Trier's final nihilistic refusal to give his apocalyptic narrative the usual hopeful remainder."[36] Pascal is not an accidental allusion, but depending on one's predisposition and intellectual preferences, one could also draw in Schopenhauer, as Shaviro does. As I remarked in the chapter on Houellebecq, these are the obligatory heroes, the *usual suspects* within the philosophical tradition of pessimism, as well as speculative realism. Is the ending of *Melancholia* not, by that very logic, the perfect example of what Schopenhauer calls a *nihil negativum*: An annihilation of a world, which is already *nothing*? An abolition of a will that is a void to begin with; a will to nothing, a will of nothing? As Schopenhauer concludes in *The World as Will and Representation*: "What remains after the complete abolition of the Will is, for all who are full of the Will, assuredly nothing (*Nichts*). But also conversely, to those in whom the Will has turned and denied itself, this very real world of ours with all its suns and galaxies, is – nothing."[37] Do we not witness something similar in von Trier's movie: A negation of a negation which does not bring about a beautiful Hegelian *Aufhebung*, but merely transposes the nothingness to a higher order, a nothingness to the nth degree?

This kind of reading would imply that the planet Melancholia affirms and finally realizes the dream that Justine has been entertaining all along (a depressive's dream about death, about the end of everything that is), or, rather, that it confirms the Nothing which she has not only *imagined* but *incarnated*: The emptiness of time that can be said to be depression's *Eigenzeit*. For her part, Justine plans (her only plan!) to give the planet a warm welcome, as she lies by the creek, completely naked, bathing in its fluorescent blue light while masturbating, in an orgiastic scene witnessed by her horrified sister. If she has any desire left, it seems to be inextricably bound up with the planet's desire for destruction. As she later says to her sister: "The earth is evil. We don't need to grieve for it," and "nobody will miss it." For all its inevitability, the end of the world or the loss of the future is thus more than a *fact;* it is precisely also a *fantasy*. Does the closing spectacle, the planetary collision, not function as the perfection and fulfillment of Justine's apocalyptic fantasies? Is this not what von Trier wants his characters and his viewers to see when they have stopped blinking: That the Earth is evil and there is no reason to grieve for it; that the world ends and so much the better, the sooner the better. Is this not the cosmic pessimism and depressive cynicism, embodied by Justine and expressed by the movie?

No.

Scene 4. An eschatological optimism against all evidence to the contrary

Something happens in the ultimate, or penultimate, scene of *Melancholia*. Something that should give one cause to pause for a moment and reconsider the seemingly evident interpretation of Justine as a figure of depressive cynicism, and the film itself as a harbinger of cosmic, speculative pessimism. Despite the fact that Justine has unyieldingly refused to grieve for the Earth, or to participate in her sister's plan to sit on the terrace with a glass of red wine and wait for the end of the world, Justine does not do nothing. Despite what the movie otherwise sets the stage for, what Lars von Trier's inclinations may usually be, and what Justine herself has hitherto expressed, she leaves cynicism, nihilism and pessimism behind. She abandons the position that emanates a tense and obstinate *whatever*. Instead she takes care of her nephew and together they build "a magic cave" whose architectural structure can perhaps best be described as a provisional and porous tipi made out of wood. This is how they face the end of the world. In my view, this gesture on Justine's part is an act of radical hope and optimism, however paradoxical – an act not to be mistaken for escapism, Buddhist bliss or an inner freedom gained at the expense of the outer world. It is not an eschatology of resurrection but a reparative and fabulative eschatology, oriented toward the future rather than the past, toward the future of things rather than the end of all things. As Ernst Bloch writes in *The Principle of Hope*: "True genesis is not at the beginning but at the end."[38]

Suicide in the stable or a glass of wine on the terrace?

Any reading of *Melancholia* that lets itself be dazzled by the notion of a world-without-us, of a thing-in-itself, and of an inhuman objectivity, risks forgetting that what the movie is really occupied with is the (inter)subjective and bodily responses of the characters to the crisis they are facing. Instead of emphasizing the importance of abandoning an *all too human perspective*, the second part of the movie is a study of the various ways in which the different characters deal with the disaster: The (end of the) world *for us*.

During the evening everything seems to be fine, and Claire is in a state of relative calm, falling asleep outside in a garden chair. But the next morning something is wrong: John panics, jotting down notes, making calculations by the telescope, knowing full well that the fly-by is – and perhaps was all along – an illusion. This is the last we see of him alive. Claire wakes up and, using the gauge device described above, discovers the truth. Panicking, she searches frantically for John and eventually she finds him in the stable, dead beside the horses; he has taken the pills that she bought earlier, just in case.

In a very conscious and concise way, the film presents several models for action following the characters' realization that the planet Melancholia plans to stay on course and crash into planet Earth. John, the man of natural science, is the first to crack: He who preached to his wife that everything was going to be okay, that she needed to stay calm and at all costs refrain from doing anything stupid like killing herself, is precisely the one who commits suicide first, because he cannot face the prospect of the planetary collision. Neither can Claire for that matter, who has been all too dependent on her husband's soothing tales of scientific validity. When these are undermined by the course of events, her only wish is to sit on the porch and drink a glass of red wine with her sister and son. She wants them to spend the remaining time together, "to do it the right way." However, this plan is not well received by Justine. Enjoying some decadent bourgeois pleasures when the end is near? No thank you. How about a song, Beethoven's Ninth, something like that? Justine sarcastically inquires of her sister, and in fact this is exactly what Claire wants:

> Justine: You want to meet on the terrace, and sip wine, the three of us?
> Claire: It would make me happy.
> Justine: Do you know what I think of your plan?
> Claire: No. I was hoping you might like it.
> Justine: I think it's a piece of shit.
> Claire: Please, Justine. I just want it to be nice…
> Justine: Nice? Why don't we meet on the fucking toilet?

This is the point at which Justine is beginning to remind everyone of her mother, who left the wedding early and does not cherish any illusions whatsoever. The mother is the perfect cynic. So, usually, is Lars von Trier, especially in his movie *Antichrist*. When Justine declares that everything tastes like ashes, or that the Earth is evil and no one will miss it, it seems like a perfect example of depressive cynicism. Except that this is not where Justine or the movie *Melancholia* ends. At the last moment the plot and character deviate from this trajectory and the logic that the director had otherwise ruthlessly set up. One must therefore avoid the seduction of these kinds of refrains, so typical of Lars von Trier: Life is evil, chaos reigns, nothing matters anymore, everything amounts to something merely akin to playing the violin as the ship goes down.

After having realized what is happening, Leo is absolutely terrified and approaches Justine. "Dad says there's nothing to do then. Nowhere to hide," he says. Justine replies: "If your dad said that, then he's forgotten about something. He's forgotten about the magic cave." They go to look for some pieces of wood with which to build the "magic cave," and are sitting right there in it as the world and the movie come to an end. But how to read this final scene if it is not an instance of von Trier sadistically toying with his viewers, tempting us to sustain yet another silly fantasy? If he is not mocking us for being so stupid and naïve as to believe that there was any hope left?

The paranoid vs. the reparative, the shelter vs. the tipi

In the essay "Paranoid Reading and Reparative Reading, or, You're So Paranoid, You Probably Think This Essay Is About You," Eve Kosofsky Sedgwick develops a useful distinction between paranoid and reparative practice. Wanting to achieve total clarity and certainty about future events, the paranoid mode, according to Sedgwick, shuts out any kind of unpredictability, uncertainty and contingency. A paranoid person wants first and foremost to avoid surprises, and thus lives in close proximity to a sense of the inevitable. This person prefers to be *right* rather than *redeemed*. It is more unacceptable and unwanted for something to be "unanticipated" than "unchallenged."[39] The reparative is an alternative model and closely related to depression, to what Sedgwick – with Melanie Klein – calls the depressive "position." This position is not only the place for a dissolution of the self but for a potential reparation as well, insofar as the depressive – as opposed to the paranoid – position is not based, and does not rely, on suspicious delusions or projections of pure hate. It is characterized by a different set of affects, an ambivalence of love *and* hate, and is not completely alien to the experience that it is, or can become, possible to "repair" one's fraught relationship with one's self, with reality and its various subjects and objects.

The fundamental divergence between the two positions or practices can be perceived as two very different futurologies: What Sedgwick conceives as "the unidirectionally future-oriented vigilance of paranoia" versus the more multi-directional future-orientation of the depressive position.[40] The closed circuit of the alert and cautious mode of paranoia versus the more open and porous state of depression. Necessity versus contingency.

The paranoid gaze is one of inevitability and fatalism, a gaze sparkling with necessity: It is meant to be like this; it has to be like this; it cannot be any different. What is, is absolutely necessary. The plan, no matter how dramatic or destructive, must be taken to its ultimate limit. Conversely, the depressive and reparative gaze is not as rigid in terms of time and temporality, nor as afraid of what might happen. It is more gentle, flexible, even naïve, but this also implies that there is less comfort in the depressive position, since it is not characterized by the absolute certainty that marks and comforts every paranoid person. As Mark Fisher writes (in a context that has nothing to do with this one except for the relation between depression and paranoia): "The depressive cannot even lay claim to the comforts that a paranoiac can enjoy, since he cannot believe that the strings are pulled by any one. No flow, no connectivity in the depressive's nervous system."[41]

A comparison might be useful here: In Jeff Nichols' movie *Take Shelter* (2011), the protagonist Curtis (Michael Shannon) is a paranoid-schizophrenic whose apocalyptic visions – of a kind of motor oil rain falling from the sky – turn out in the end to be true. In the meantime, before his visions have been collaborated by reality, he takes every precautionary measure to ensure that he and his family will be safe when the disaster arrives. He thus buys a container and builds a shelter in his backyard, buried underground in an attempt to make it impenetrable and totally bulletproof. He is thus a paranoid who acts accordingly. In terms of structural engineering, the contrast with *Melancholia* could not be starker; affect and architecture go hand in hand. In *Take Shelter*, Curtis – just like John in *Melancholia* – cannot live in a world where everything is not determined in advance. He wants no surprises, takes no chances and does not want to be unprepared. He is a survivalist prepper. This is why he builds a tight shelter underground, whereas Justine constructs a transparent and provisional tipi on the top of a hill. Her final reparative act, which emerges from her depressive position, is thus more attuned to the precariousness of the relations in and of life, more open toward what Sedgwick calls the "the heartbeat of contingency."[42]

Contingency, however, is not a given. As Sedgwick draws our attention to, contingency is a continuous work. In relation to *Melancholia* the obvious question is: Which contingency? The world is undeniably coming to an end, Melancholia arrives, the disaster occurs, there is no doubt about it. But in the movie, reparation takes the form of a fabulation. The condition for confronting and countering the catastrophe is not knowledge but belief. In *Melancholia,* this is what John realizes too late: In a dangerous or potentially lethal situation, science is not enough; knowledge alone is insufficient. Something irrational is needed, an illusion of some kind. Although Justine prides herself on knowing things, we should not, as viewers, see her as a melancholic who is necessarily in possession of some secret and special knowledge. This would be a paranoid logic, and in a sense science generally operates in a *paranoid* way as its entire edifice is built on the need to know all. This is the direction in which most readings of *Melancholia* go: Sandberg – who only allots a few words to Justine's depression – refers to her as "a mystic depressive," "the one with special depressive vision."[43] Shaviro, who does assign some attention to the phenomenon of depression in his superb article, writes that she "just sees things as they actually are."[44] What these rather romantic ideas of a depressive realism – often inspired by Freud's assessment that the depressed or melancholic person had "a keener eye for the truth than others who are not melancholic"[45] – tend to forget or overlook is that any real act requires a speculative *as if*. As Nietzsche remarks in *The Birth of Tragedy,* knowledge kills action. Belief or illusions, on the other hand, resuscitate the possibility of action. It is vital to act *as if* the worst that can happen has in fact already happened in an attempt to avoid the inevitable outcome.[46] Is this not Justine's *modus operandi*? As Claire says to her sister at one point: "You have it easy, don't you? You just imagine the worst thing possible."

This is in fact precisely what Justine is doing, though not in order to fall back into the comforting pillows of cynical pessimism, where the lack of illusion dictates that nothing really matters anymore, so one might as well do exactly nothing on the very last day.[47] Nor does she imagine the worst in order to overreact in a paranoid fashion (what paranoia and pessimism share is a state of absolute certainty, but while the paranoid tends to overreact on the basis of that certainty, the pessimist does not act at all). As argued, the final scene in *Melancholia* unequivocally refuses this interpretation. Justine imagines the worst thing possible – the one thing she is able to imagine – and *then* acts by fabricating a myth, which takes the form of a declaration of love. It is as though the depressive's imaginarium is specifically suited to perform this task. Nothing could be easier, in this state of mind and being, than to regard the future as a thing of the past and imminent events as foregone conclusions. Openness toward contingency is, in a sense, necessarily depressive, insofar as depression is permeated by a recognition of the precariousness and perishability of all things within a subjective, objective and cosmic horizon.

Justine's final fabulation/reparation – the tipi – is of course an illusion. But as von Trier seems to say, it is a necessary illusion even if the world ends; or rather, because it ends. It is necessary to have something to believe in, because belief does not sabotage but supports the transcendental conditions of any given practice. To quote Wallace Stevens' *Adagia* again: "The final belief is to believe in a fiction, which you know to be a fiction, there being nothing else. The exquisite truth is to know that it is a fiction and that you believe it willingly."[48] In contrast to those critics, for whom this act by Justine is illusory and thus useless, I would contend, and in what follows conclude, that the fabrication of the "magic cave" is useful precisely insofar as it is illusory.[49]

Radical hope, utopian realism

In this sense, the movie instantiates a version of the kind of radical hope described by Jonathan Lear in *Radical Hope* – a book whose cover is illustrated with a tipi very similar to the one in *Melancholia*. The context for Lear's book is the cultural devastation faced by the Crow Native American tribe around the end of the nineteenth century. Interviewing the former chief Plenty Coups, Lear writes that he "would like to consider hope as it might arise at one of the limits of human existence [...] What makes this hope *radical* is that it is directed toward a future goodness that transcends the current ability to understand what it is."[50] As Bonnie Honig points out in a reading that compares Lear's concept of radical hope with von Trier's *Melancholia*, it is clear that:

> Justine's magic cave will not "work," not if surviving catastrophic collision is the aim [...] And, indeed, we gain a new perspective on Plenty Coups, with von Trier's help, because in Justine's ritual, the aim is clearly not survival [...] Justine, Claire, and maybe even Leo all know these twigs and branches would not protect them from world destruction. And yet at the same time, building the magic cave is not just a going through the motions either [...] The importance of this flimsy little structure at the end of the film may be signaled by its absence from an earlier sequence, at the beginning of the film.[51]

What *Melancholia* offers is "an anti-teleological rendition of hope,"[52] in that it is a hope based on contingency rather than teleology; a hope that it is not rooted in any idea of a time *after* the apocalypse, or in the dream of a hereafter succeeding the catastrophe. Nor is it a hope that goes from the present to the future, since the future is not the object of hope – nor its effect – but its cause; it is hope as a temporal loop, even if only for a split second before extinction.

The hope activated at the end of *Melancholia* is even more radical than that in Lear's book, since the destruction that Justine and her family face is not so much cultural as biological. Their situation is beyond any doubt, objectively hopeless. But as Søren Kierkegaard writes in *Sickness unto Death,* hope is most relevant when "a person is brought to his extremity, when humanly speaking, there is no possibility."[53] The hope in *Melancholia* is, in a word, hope by virtue of the absurd.

Emerging – not in spite of the fact but – because we are at the end, this radical hope could even be considered a specific form of optimism. In his trilogy *The Principle of Hope,* whose main focus is an eschatological "not yet" (*noch nicht*), which opens a horizon of expectation in the midst of the elimination of expectation as such, Ernst Bloch lays out the key to the whole project on the very page: "It is a question of learning hope."[54] At the end of the first volume of his trilogy Bloch mentions the term "artificially conditioned optimism" ("künstlich bedingter Optimismus"), distinguishing it both from "unconditional pessimism" ("bedingungsloser Pessimismus") and "rotten optimism" ("faulen Optimismus"). In his characteristically poetic style, Bloch writes:

Unconditional pessimism [...] promotes the business of reaction not much less than artificially conditioned optimism; the latter is nevertheless not so stupid that it does not believe in anything at all. It does not immortalize the trudging of the little life, does not give the humanity the face of a chloroformed gravestone. It does not give the world the deathly sad background in front of which it is not worth doing anything at all.[55]

For Bloch, this artificially conditioned optimism could transform into a "critical-militant optimism" ("kritischmilitanter Optimismus") and was in any case preferable to unconditional pessimism precisely because it does not work as an anesthetic; it does not function as a cloth soaked in chloroform; it is not a pretext for doing nothing.

This kind of optimism has little to do with what Lauren Berlant calls cruel optimism, or with what Lovecraft, in a blunter manner, calls bland or smirking optimism. It is not the optimism that underpins the ideology of happiness, as exposed by Barbara Ehrenreich, and according to which Justine's depression and unhappiness is immoral, a failure of will, or even a secret will. Rather, it is an optimism *conditioned by* the recognition that things really *are* bad, that the times are dire and the end is alarmingly near; it is an optimism that does not ignore or repress the misery and suffering in the world.[56] As Bloch writes: "[P]essimism is paralysis per se, whereas even the most rotten optimism can still be the stupefaction from which there is an awakening."[57]

Let us not forget the biographical and historical circumstances: It was in a wretched exile in the US (Bloch and his wife, Karola, had no choice but to flee Germany at the end of the 1930s), between 1938 and 1947, that Bloch wrote *The Principle of Hope,* although it was not published until 1954-1959 in the former DDR.[58] In short, he wrote it during the Second World War, while receiving news of Hitler causing havoc on the other side of the Atlantic, of Karola's parents being deported to a concentration camp, and of Walter Benjamin, Bloch's lifelong friend, dying in the Pyrenees at the border between Spain and France in 1940. Still he wrote a book about hope. Not despite but rather because of the horror of the historical present.

In fact, this principle of hope – or utopian impulse – is what endows *Melancholia* with a certain realism. Instead of subscribing to the romantic notion of depressive realism – Justine as the one who knows, who sees things how they really are – a reading of *Melancholia* would benefit from following Bloch even further, to say that there can be no realism worthy of the name without a certain element of utopia. What is at stake are not the realistic qualities of utopian endeavors but, conversely, the utopian dimension of realism proper.[59] This claim is supported by Jürgen Moltmann, who in *Theology of Hope* points out it is conventional realism – "the celebrated realism of the stark facts" – that is utopian, which is to say unrealistic, while utopian hope alone is realistic.[60] This could be the radical and paradoxical lesson of Lars von Trier's movie.

Melancholia would then be a movie that leads nowhere, except perhaps to a kind of hope. The image that thus remains after everything has ended, the screen has gone black and Wagner's music has abated, is an image of a miniature of humanity that is heading for that moment when everything seems to be moving toward the end, and yet also toward a new beginning of some kind. It is an image of the last humans, who at the edge of total collapse are reconciled in an act of cosmic reparation. However, for Bloch it was all-important to really realize utopian dreams and hopes; the essential content of hope is not hope, he wrote.[61] Potentialities are not enough in the end, as an end in themselves; imaginary solutions to real problems are not gateways to utopia. But in *Melancholia*, we do not get any realization of hope – which is not to say that the outcome is irrelevant, but that faith and hope do not depend on it – though we do get the gesture, the impulse, and a provisional yet real and concrete image of what Bloch called an "architecture of hope."[62] We get more than "stark facts," and more than a chloroformed version of being; we get the utopianism of the not-yet, the realism of the maybe-not.

Smile and die: The paradoxically happy end of melancholia (Threshold)

In *Melancholia,* Justine's depression takes the form of a deepening sense of alienation from the other guests at the wedding, her family and her husband. What separates Justine from all the other guests is that, whereas all of them take part in a bourgeois futurological game, Justine is the only one who does not constantly plan ahead, anticipate what is going to happen in the near or distant future, or project hopes and expectations into the not-yet. In one shot, she sits motionless in the background, while the other guests dance in the foreground, indicating a sharply delineated desynchronization between individual and society, and a stark juxtaposition of two temporal orders. She sits, staring into the nothingness that is not only in front of her but deep within, tearing her apart from the inside out. As Wittgenstein once wrote: "The world of the happy is quite different from the world of the unhappy."

The abyss between the frantic, futurological activity of the environment and Justine's complete lack thereof, reveals more than the nature of Justine's "illness"; it gives us an insight into a particular idea of the "healthy" individual. The healthy individual is one who is able to plan ahead in order to maximize his or her (feeling of) happiness. In *Melancholia,* happiness is a moral imperative imposed upon Justine from every side. What is at stake, so the movie seems to suggest, is something greater than Justine's individual life. At stake is sociality as such. Every tiny moment of unhappiness and every sign of depression is an intrusion in the social order, a violation of the moral regime. In the eyes of the other characters, her happiness is not a matter of objective circumstances, genetic dispositions or external factors, but solely a matter of Justine's own choice. As Coca Cola declares in one of their latest, importunate campaigns:

"Choose happiness." Obviously, Justine is in no position to choose that, but she does try to put a good face on it. She knows she is perceived as a "bad person" – to use Zupančič's phrase once again – because she feels bad, because she is unhappy and depressed. So she smiles and she smiles and she smiles. Smile or die? Smile and die.

But then the planet Melancholia comes, and everything and everyone are about to vanish from the face of the Earth. At first glance this only seems to confirm Justine's almost masturbatory masochism, fulfilling her apocalyptic fantasies and her longing for the end of everything. But as we have seen, it is not that simple. In the end, Justine does not fall back into a state of comforting cynicism, nor does she indulge in what could be called the illusion of illusionlessness. But this is not where Justine or the movie ends. The end result is not cosmic pessimism nor is it a cynical and capitalist version of depressive realism. The realism in question is one of a different kind, a realism based on what could be rather than on what is. Even though Justine has called her sister's plan to drink a last glass of wine on the terrace "a piece of shit," and totally refused to build castles in the air (not literally, of course), she takes part in a final act of illusion as she builds a "magic cave" on the top of the hill where she, her nephew and her sister can face annihilation together. Refusing, in the last instance, to abandon the realm of illusions, Justine thus engages in an act of reparation in the form of a fabulation. In a sense there is a strange similarity between Lars von Trier and David Foster Wallace, in that both artists accentuate a reparative and fabulative practice as a way out of depression. The crucial point of divergence is that in von Trier's movie, this practice assumes a wholly different cosmological if not eschatological dimension. In my anti-romantic and anti-pessimist reading – is pessimism not the ultimate romantic attitude? – the "intention" of *Melancholia* is not to confront the characters or the audience with the pure void, the ultimate horror vacui, or the world-without-us, but to erect a principle of hope which only becomes relevant when there is none; a hope that emerges at the horizon of pure hopelessness, or even at the prospect of the end of the world. In this reading, the end – despite von Trier's promise or warning that he has done away with such things – does indeed become a happy ending.

Epilogue (three songs and three paradoxes)

"Clap along if you feel like a room without a roof," sings Pharrell Williams on the monster hit "Happy" from 2014. The tune is relevant in this context, not only because it enounces, spontaneously and quite unabashedly, the contemporary ideology of happiness in a sing-along refrain and to a dance-able beat, but more importantly because it gives an outline of the architectural counter-image to depression. Depression is not a room without a roof but, on the contrary, a room without a floor; a fall into a never-ending abyss, a bottomless bottom. There is nothing to break the fall, no ground to stop, much less soften the fall. Alternatively, there is a sense in which there is always a bottom below, as Malvina Reynolds sings in the song with the telling title "There's a bottom below" (1970): "Do you think you've hit bottom?/ Do you think you've hit bottom?/ Oh, no/ There's a bottom below/ There's a low below the low you know/ You can't imagine how far you can go down." In depression, there is indeed a low below the low you know. So naturally, one does not clap along. One does not get up, but stays in bed. Exit Pharrell, enter Le Tigre: "Do you wanna stay in bed all day? (yeah)/ Do you remember feeling any other way? (no)." In reality, though, depression in this book is not understood in spatial or architectural, but temporal terms. Even if depression defies definitive definitions, one can say that depression is a temporal pathology: That the time of depression is a time outside time.

Depression can thus be characterized as a desynchronized rhythm, or more specifically, by a sense of futurelessness that is both personal and political. I suggest that depression is the (pathological) feeling that history has come to an end, that the future is closed off, frozen once and for all. A present that has aborted all futures – could it not be said by now that this inversion of Leibniz's dictum – that the present is pregnant with the future – captures the temporality of depression, its hopelessness, its futurelessness?

This is in any case what the works of Michel Houellebecq, David Foster Wallace, Claire Fontaine and Lars von Trier – for all their differences – illustrate. In their respective anatomizations of depression these artists share an orientation toward the future rather than the past. What some of their works also show is that the problem relating to and resonating with the phenomenon of depression is not that we are separated from our selves, each other, our work and our life in general. The problem is not one of anomie, nor of the pulverization of social bonds; this is, at most, an epiphenomenal problem. Rather, these works tell us that the core of the problem of alienation is proximity rather than distance; the total integration of work and life rather than a brutal separation between the two; a "warm" affective economy rather than a cold and abstract one. To repeat the line from Andrew Solomon's *Noonday Demon* that functions as a kind of refrain in this book: "We are depressed not because we are so far removed from what we want, but because we are merged with it."

Three pertinent paradoxes have furthermore been at work in the works analyzed: The paradoxical existence of depressive art as such; the paradoxical comedy of depressive art; and, the paradoxical hope sometimes made manifest in depressive art.

The first paradox is that such a thing as depressive art even exists. In itself it approaches a contradiction in terms. The depressed person experiences a complete lack of creativity and imagination, denying an artist the very tools of his or her trade. This could be called the constitutive aporia of depressive literature and art: Strictly speaking, the depressive person does not write (or paint, or compose, or...). Thus, the question is not only how depression becomes a problem *of* literature and art in general, but also how depression at the same time becomes a problem *for* literature and art.

The second paradox has to do with a dark variety of comedy that arises in depressive art. Søren Kierkegaard has written that "the melancholy have the best sense of the comic."[1] In fact, Kierkegaard repeatedly states, in his *Concluding Unscientific Postscript*, that a mis-relation or contradiction lies at the root of the comic, and therefore the comic is everywhere in so far as life is essentially characterized by contradiction. Thus, Kierkegaard arrives at a strikingly simple law of the comic and the law is: "Where there is life, there is contradiction, and wherever there is contradiction, the comic is present."[2] In other words: A mis-relation in the self, or a de-synchronization between self and world, not only forms the basis of deep despair; it is also the stuff that comedy is made of. The structure is, in a way, the same.

The third paradox relates to the fact that the depressive scenes sometimes evidence, however briefly, a paradoxical impulse of optimism and hope. In the words of Lauren Berlant, they can be said to unfold an "interregnum of hesitation when the relation of living to a fantasy of life has to be reinvented."[3] There is a quasi-dialectical relation between despair and hope; between depression and utopia. When the tyrant Bane, in the Batman film *The Dark Knight Rises*, states that there can be no despair without hope, I want to add that there can be no hope without despair either. As Jürgen Moltmann writes in his book *The Theology of Hope,* which together with Ernst Bloch's *The Principle of Hope* has been a great source of inspiration for these particular reflections and for my reading of Lars von Trier's *Melancholia,* despair presupposes hope – and vice versa. "The pain of despair surely lies in the fact that a hope is there, but no way opens up towards its fulfillment," Moltmann writes.[4] The proper eschatological question according to him is the one once formulated by Kant: What may I hope for? But this question is inextricable from and concomitant with a second: Of what may I, or should I despair? These two questions are, in a sense, one and the same. Perhaps depression, or depressive art, is able to show us an alternative to the dead end-dualism of escapism or maintenance of the *status quo*; between what Bloch calls rotten optimism and unconditional pessimism. Given the choice of the two, Bloch opted for optimism, given that it is not so stupid "that it does not believe in anything at all. It does not immortalize the trudging of the little life, does not give humanity the face of a chloroformed gravestone."[5] However, if one has spent a long time living in a malevolent and hopeless state of depression, it is undoubtedly the case, to quote William Faulkner's *Light in August,* that "the machinery for hoping requires more than twenty-four hours to get started, to get into motion again."

Endnotes

Parts of chapter 2 have been published as the article "Finding the un-lovable object lovable – empathy and depression in David Foster Wallace" in *Studies in American Fiction*, Vol. 45 (1), 2018, while portions of chapter 4 have been printed in Danish under the title "Depression og/eller apokalypse: Lars von Trier's *Melancholia*" in the journal *K.&K.*, Vol 120, 2015.

Prologue (two questions)

1. Édouard Levé, *Suicide*, trans. Jan Steyn (Champaign: Dalkey Archive Press, 2011), pp. 38-39.

Introduction. Welcome to the world's happiest nation

1. Allan V. Horwitz and Jerome Wakefield, *The Loss of Sadness: How Psychiatry Transformed Normal Sorrow Into Depressive Disorder* (Oxford: Oxford University Press, 2007), p. 25.

2. Christine Ross, The Aesthetics of Disengagement: *Contemporary Art and Depression* (Minneapolis: University of Minnesota Press, 2006), p. xvii.

3. Karl Jaspers, *General Psychopathology*, trans. J. Hoenig and Marian Hamilton (Manchester: Manchester University Press, 1963), p. 84.

4. Ibid., p. 86.

5. In fact, the DSM relies on a definition of depression as a mood or affective disorder. I agree with the wording of the definition but not with its content. Perhaps depression is indeed an affective disorder, or a mood disorder, but the question is: how does that affective or mood disorder feel? What is the affect of the affective disorder, so to speak? This is just one of the reasons I do not subscribe to the definition to be found in the DSM. A more fundamental problem is the reductive and rather old-fashioned

understanding of mood and affect informing the DSM: The tendency to de-contextualize moods and affects, to rely on the ancient dualism of body and mind/brain, to pathologize certain emotional responses and so on. Theoretically this book is therefore more in line not only with Jaspers, but recent affect theory, whose insights and attainments are overall able to nuance, supplement and complicate the definition of depression as a mood or affect disorder presented in the DSM. One of the cornerstones of affect theory, taken somewhat misleadingly as a whole, is firstly that feelings and affects must be taken seriously, and secondly that affects are as much collective, social and political phenomena as they are psychological, private and individual. Crucial reference points in this regard are Ann Cvetkovich's *Depression: A Public Feeling* and Lauren Berlant's *Cruel Optimism*. Furthermore, affect theory often seeks to depathologize negative feelings of sadness and unhappiness, thereby, as Ann Cvetkovich writes, granting questions like "How do I feel?" or "How does capitalism feel?" a real legitimacy (Ann Cvetkovich, *Depression: A Public Feeling* (Durham: Duke University Press, 2012), p. 3). As Cvetkovich also writes: "Depression, or alternative accounts of what gets called depression, is thus a way to describe neoliberalism and globalization, or the current state of political economy, in affective terms." (Ibid., 11).

6. Thomas Fuchs, "Implicit and Explicit Temporality," in *Philosophy, Psychiatry, & Psychology* 12 (3), 2005, p. 196.

7. See: Martin Wyllie, "Lived time and psychopathology," in *Philosophy, Psychiatry, & Psychology*, Volume 12, Number 3, 2005; Mette Rønberg, "At se sig selv i fremtiden: Erfaringer med en depressionsdiagnose," in *Diagnoser. Perspektiver, kritik og diskussion*, ed. Svend Brinkmann and Anders Petersen (København: Forlaget Klim, 2015); David A. Karp, *Speaking of Sadness. Depression, Disconnection, and the*

Meanings of Illness (Oxford: Oxford University Press, 1996).

8. Frederick T. Melges, *Time and the Inner Future. A Temporal Approach to Psychiatric Disorders* (New York: John Wiley & Sons, Inc, 1982), p. 178.

9. Franco "Bifo" Berardi, *After the Future*, trans. Arianna Bove et al. (Chico: AK Press, 2011), p. 126.

10. Franco "Bifo" Berardi, *The Uprising: On Poetry and Finance* (Los Angeles: Semiotext(e), 2012), p. 100.

11. Berardi, *After the Future*, p. 59.

12. Mark Fisher, *Capitalist Realism* (London: Zero Books, 2009), p. 2.

13. Mark Fisher, *Ghosts of My Life. Writings on Depression, Hauntology and Lost Futures* (London: Zero Books, 2014), p. 27.

14. Fisher, *Capitalist Realism*, p. 5.

15. Sigmund Freud, "Mourning and Melancholia," in *On Murder, Mourning and Melancholia*, trans. Shaun Whiteside (London: Penguin Books, 2005), p. 206.

16. Fredric Jameson, *A Singular Modernity: Essay on the Ontology of the Present* (London/New York: Verso, 2002), p. 29.

17. I use the concept neoliberalism as Philip Mirowski defines it in a critical displacement of Michel Foucault's groundbreaking work (Philip Mirowski, *Never Let a Serious Crisis Go to Waste: How Neoliberalism Survived the Financial Meltdown* (London/New York: Verso, 2013), pp. 53ff.). Neoliberalism is thus not only understood as an ideological or even idealistic concept, developed by a few visionary thinkers at the Mont Pelerin Society from 1947 onwards and then put to work and realized in the years to come. As the current form of global capitalism, neoliberalism is an economic and political concept and system that has as its primary goal "the restoration of class power" (David Harvey, *A Brief History of Neoliberalism* (Oxford: Oxford University Press, 2007), p. 16). At the same time,

however, neoliberalism also entails a certain production of subjectivity (an insight which admittedly must be attributed to Foucault): A production or modulation of the self as innovative and entrepreneurial, perhaps best captured by the concept of human capital.

18. Wolfgang Streeck, *Buying Time: The Delayed Crisis of Democratic Capitalism* (London/New York: Verso, 2014), 165.

19. Michel Houellebecq, *The Possibility of an Island*, trans. Gavin Bowd (New York: Vintage International, 2007), p. 337.

20. Andrew Solomon, *The Noonday Demon. An Atlas of Depression* (New York: Scribner, 2001), p. 326.

21. It is, however, not the *only* story about alienation: I am making no universalizing claims. The story I am telling is one about a specific form of alienation in the Western world, in which alienated subjects are not excluded on the basis of their race, gender, class etc., but rather included and inscribed in the web of neoliberal capitalism – until the very moment of pathological collapse.

22. Alain Ehrenberg, *The Weariness of the Self. Diagnosing the History of Depression in the Contemporary Age*, trans. Enrico Caouette et al. (Montréal: Mcgill-Queen's University Press, 2010), p. 43.

23. Bernard Stiegler, *Uncontrollable Societies of Disaffected Individuals. Disbelief and Discredit, Volume 2*, trans. Daniel Ross (Cambridge: Polity Press, 2013), p. 12.

24. In his book *The Soul at Work,* Berardi writes: "This is just what we need today: An awareness of depression that would not be depressing" (Franco "Bifo" Berardi, *The Soul at Work* (Cambridge: MIT Press, 2009), p. 134). Along the same lines Ann Cvetkovich states: "The concept of political depression is not, it should be emphasized, meant to be wholly depressing." (Cvetkovich, *Depression: A Public Feeling,* p. 2).

25.   Lauren Berlant, "Starved," in *South Atlantic Quarterly* 106 (3), 2007, p. 434.

Chapter 1. The future was empty – Michel Houellebecq

1.   Michel Houellebecq, *Whatever*, trans. Paul Hammond (London: Serpent's Tail, 2011), pp. 134-135.
2.   Houellebecq, *Whatever*, p. 38.
3.   Michel Houellebecq, *The Possibility of an Island* (New York: Vintage International, 2007), p. 32.
4.   Houellebecq, *Whatever*, p. 131.
5.   Søren Kierkegaard, *Sickness unto Death*, ed. and trans. Howard V. Hong and Edna H. Hong (Princeton: Princeton University Press, 1980), p. 36; 39.
6.   Ibid., p. 71.
7.   Ibid., p. 15.
8.   Ibid.
9.   Ibid.
10.   Houellebecq, *Whatever*, p. 135.
11.   A few thinkers have elaborated on the idea that existential or spiritual despair can be regarded as a central component of depression, a kind of isotope. Karl Jaspers – who found a great source of inspiration in Kierkegaard – is not the only writer to have devoted some attention to the relation between depression and despair. In his book *On Depression. Drugs, Diagnosis, and Despair in the Modern World,* Nassir Ghaemi places quite an emphasis on this particular relation, and Ann Cvetkovich seeks "a model for thinking about depression as a spiritual problem" in her book *Depression: A Public Feeling* (Cvetkovich, *Depression: A Public Feeling,* p. 24). The Kierkegaardian notion of despair is one such model, I would argue. Of course, this does not mean that depression can be reduced to a spiritual problem but that the notion of spiritual despair can expand and supplement existing explications of depression.

12. Fisher, *Ghosts of My Life*, p. 59.
13. H. P. Lovecraft, *The Road to Madness* (New York: Del Rey, 1996), p. 59.
14. Houellebecq, *Whatever*, p. 82
15. Fisher, *Ghosts of My Life*, pp. 60-61.
16. Jonathan Franzen, *How to be Alone* (London: 4th Estate, 2002), p. 87.
17. Freud, "Mourning and Melancholia," p. 206.
18. See for instance Ben Jeffery's brilliant little book *Anti-Matter*, which explicitly draws upon the notion of depressive realism, or Paul Berman's review of *Atomised* in *New Republic* from 2000, which bears the simple title "Depressive Lucidity," a phrase that turns up in the novel. Implicitly, the same idea flourishes in a sociological reading like Anders Petersen and Michael Hviid Jacobsen's "Houellebecq's Dystopia – A Case of the Elective Affinity between Sociology and Literature." What must be stressed is that the hypothesis of depressive realism or any other kind of romantic notion of depression must be abandoned, even if the artists or artworks themselves seem to subscribe to such ideas, as *Whatever* does at a glance. Indeed, at one point the narrator implies a connection between his wretched life and his unbending clarity of perception; he is miserable because he can see what misery life in reality consists of (Houellebecq, *Whatever*, p. 46).
19. Houellebecq, *Whatever*, pp. 13-14.
20. Ibid., p. 40.
21. Ibid., p. 3.
22. Victoria Best and Martin Crowley, *The New Pornographies. Explicit sex in recent French fiction and film* (Manchester: Manchester University Press, 2007), p. 185.
23. Ben Jeffery, *Anti-Matter: Michel Houellebecq and Depressive Realism* (London: Zero Books, 2011), p. 53.
24. Houellebecq, *The Possibility of an Island*, p. 133.

25. Bruno Latour, "On some of the affects of capitalism," lecture given at The Royal Danish Academy of Fine Arts in Copenhagen, Denmark, 2014, http://www.bruno-latour. fr/sites/default/files/136-AFFECTS-OF-K-COPENHAGUE. pdf.

26. Houellebecq, *Whatever,* p. 153.

27. Søren Kierkegaard, *Either/Or vol. 1,* ed. and trans. Howard V. Hong and Edna H. Hong (Princeton: Princeton University Press, 1987), p. 105; p. 107.

28. Houellebecq, *Whatever,* p. 155.

29. Ibid., p. 66.

30. Kierkegaard, *Sickness unto Death,* p. 18.

31. Michel Houellebecq, *Atomised,* trans. Frank Wynne (London: Vintage Books, 2001), pp. 353-354.

32. Ibid., p. 379.

33. Ibid., p. 238.

34. Ibid., p. 242.

35. Ibid., p. 139.

36. Ibid., p. 352.

37. In Mark Fisher's *Capitalist Realism* hedonia is defined as "an inability to do anything else *except* pursue pleasure." (Fisher, *Capitalist Realism,* p. 22).

38. Houellebecq, *Atomised,* pp. 135-136.

39. Ibid., pp. 252-253.

40. Ibid., p. 246.

41. Ibid., p. 81.

42. It is by now conventional analysis that the critical ideas of autonomy and emancipation instanced by the events of 1968 were quickly appropriated by capitalism and transformed into a guiding principle for the neoliberal restructuring of the economy from the late '60s/early '70s onward. See, for instance: Luc Boltanski and Eve Chiapello, *The New Spirit of Capitalism,* trans. Gregory Elliott (London/New York: Verso, 2007). For more on Houellebecq and neoliberalism,

see: Carole Sweeney, *Michel Houellebecq and the Literature of Despair* (London/New York: Bloomsbury, 2013).

43. Michel Foucault, *The Birth of Biopolitics: Lectures at the Collège de France, 1978-1979*, trans. Graham Burchell (New York: Picador, 2010), p. 226.

44. Michel Houellebecq, *Platform*, trans. Frank Wynne (New York: Random House, 2002), p. 284.

45. Sweeney, *Michel Houellebecq and the Literature of Despair*, p. 12.

46. Jean Baudrillard, *The Vital Illusion*, ed. Julia Witver (New York: Columbia University Press, 2000), p. 34.

47. Ibid., p. 35.

48. Ibid., 34 – my emphasis.

49. Ibid., p. 14.

50. Ibid., p. 15.

51. Houellebecq, *Atomised*, p. 371.

52. Baudrillard, *The Vital Illusion*, p. 7.

53. Pascal Bruckner, *Perpetual Euphoria: On the Duty to Be Happy*, trans. Steven Rendall (Princeton: Princeton University Press, 2010), 219. Incidentally Bruckner – whose thoughts on happiness will become relevant in the chapter on Trier's *Melancholia* – is quoted in *Submission*.

54. Foucault, *The Birth of Biopolitics*, p. 228.

55. Mirowski, *Never Let a Serious Crisis Go to Waste*, p. 154 – my emphasis.

56. Foucault quoted in: Mirowski, *Never Let a Serious Crisis Go to Waste*, p. 105.

57. Houellebecq, *Atomised*, p. 377.

58. Houellebecq, *The Possibility of an Island*, p. 328

59. Ibid., p. 170.

60. Ibid., p. 258.

61. Ibid., p. 312.

62. Ibid., p. 305.

63. H. P. Lovecraft, *At the Mountains of Madness* (New York:

Random House, 2005), p. 15.

64. Charles Baxter, "The Hideous Unknown of H. P. Lovecraft," in *The New York Review of Books,* Vol. 61, No. 20, December 18, 2014.

65. Houellebecq, *The Possibility of an Island,* p. 328.

66. Ibid., p. 312.

67. Houellebecq, *Atomised,* p. 13.

68. Houellebecq, *The Possibility of an Island,* p. 337.

69. Ibid., pp. 325-326 – my emphasis.

70. It is of course William Faulkner ("The past is never dead. It's not even past") who lurks behind this formulation.

71. Michel Houellebecq, *Submission,* trans. Lorin Stein (London: William Heinemann, 2015), pp. 137-139. As is well known *Soumission* was published in French on the same day as the Charlie Hebdo shooting in Paris, 7 January 2015.

72. Karl Ove Knausgård, "Michel Houellebecq's 'Submission,'" in *The New York Times,* 2 November 2015, http://www.nytimes.com/2015/11/08/books/review/michel-houellebecqs-submission.html.

73. Houellebecq, *Submission,* p. 77.

74. Houellebecq, *The Possibility of an Island,* p. 165.

75. Joris-Karl Huysmans, *Against Nature,* trans. Margaret Mauldon (Oxford: Oxford University Press, 1998), pp. 179-180.

76. Huysmans, *Against Nature,* p. 178.

77. Ibid., p. 180.

78. Ibid., p. 181.

79. In a preface to *Against Nature,* written 20 years after the publication of the novel but included in my edition of it, Huysmans writes: "Indeed it does seem to be the case that nervous disorders and neuroses create fissures in the soul through which Evil may penetrate. That is an enigma which remains unexplained: the word hysteria solves nothing; it may suffice to define a physical condition, to denote an

uncontrollable turmoil of the senses, it does not account for the spiritual consequences associated with it, particularly the sins of dissimulation and falsehood which almost invariably implant themselves therein," adding, that as far as this relation between pathology and spirituality is concerned "medicine talks nonsense and theology remains silent" (Huysmans, *Against Nature*, p. 189).

80. Robert Burton, *The Anatomy of Melancholy* (New York: New York Review Books, 2001), p. 379.

81. Ibid., p. 405.

82. William James, *Writings 1902-1910* (New York: Library of America, 1988), p. 1329.

83. William James, *Varieties of Religious Experience. A Study in Human Nature* (New York: Dover Publications, 2002), p. 160.

84. Ibid., p. 161.

85. Ibid., p. 162.

86. Cf. Andrea Goulet, "Neurosyphilitics and Madmen: The French *Fin-de-siècle* Fictions of Huysmans, Lermina, and Maupassant," in *Literature, Neurology, and Neuroscience: Neurological and Psychiatric Disorders*, ed. Stanley Finger, François Boller and Anne Stiles (Amsterdam: Elsevier, 2013), pp. 73-91.

87. Houellebecq, *Submission*, p. 213.

88. Bernard-Henri Lévy and Michel Houellebecq, *Public Enemies*, trans. Miriam Frendo and Frank Wynne (New York: Random House, 2011), p. 165.

89. Houellebecq, *Submission*, p. 125.

90. Knausgård, "Michel Houellebecq's 'Submission.'"

91. As for the concept of soul or spirit, which I take to be synonymous in this context, I rely on Bernard Stiegler's concept of spirit as something individual, collective and technological, belonging to the political economy (see his works *Uncontrollable Societies of Disaffected Individuals.*

Disbelief and Discredit, Volume 2 and *The Lost Spirit of Capitalism. Disbelief and Discredit, Volume 3*) and on Franco "Bifo" Berardi's concept of soul (see his book *The Soul at Work*).

92. A theme that Houellebecq strikes time and again and also introduces at the very beginning of *Submission* (see pp. 5-6).
93. Lévy and Houellebecq, *Public Enemies*, p. 253.
94. Houellebecq, *Submission*, p. 250.
95. Houellebecq, *The Possibility of an Island*, p. 62.
96. Ibid., p. 237.
97. Gilles Deleuze and Félix Guattari, *What is Philosophy*, trans. Hugh Tomlinson and Graham Burchell (New York: Columbia University Press, 1994), p. 214.
98. Douglas Morrey, *Michel Houellebecq: Humanity and its aftermath* (Liverpool: Liverpool University Press, 2013), p. 41 – emphasis in original. (288-289).
99. Fredric Jameson, *Archaeologies of the Future. The Desire Called Utopia and Other Science Fictions* (London/New York: Verso, 2005), pp. 288-289.
100. In *Public Enemies* Houellebecq says: "I think, in dealing with humanity, it's important from time to time to take a *bacterial point of view*" (Lévy and Houellebecq, *Public Enemies*, p. 172 – italics in original), which is indeed what he does at the end of *The Map and the Territory*.
101. Houellebecq, *Platform*, p. 16.
102. Here I am paraphrasing some lines from an interview with Hungarian writer László Krasznahorkai (George Szirtes, "Interview with László Krasznahorkai," in *The White Review*, September 2013, http://www.thewhitereview.org/interviews/interview-with-laszlo-krasznahorkai/.

Chapter 2. And then nothing turned itself inside out –

David Foster Wallace

1. Stephen Burn, *Conversations with David Foster Wallace* (Jackson: University Press of Mississippi, 2012), p. 26.
2. Ibid.
3. Emmanuel Levinas, *Time and the Other*, trans. Richard A. Cohen (Pittsburgh: Duquesne University Press, 1987), p. 77.
4. David Foster Wallace, *Brief Interviews with Hideous Men* (New York: Back Bay Books, 2000), pp. 37-39.
5. Ibid., pp. 42-44.
6. Ibid., p. 44.
7. Ibid., p. 67.
8. Ibid., p. 65.
9. Ibid., p. 66.
10. Ibid.
11. Ibid., p. 68.
12. Marshall Boswell, *Understanding David Foster Wallace* (Columbia: University of South Carolina Press, 2003), p. 207.
13. Zadie Smith, *Changing my Mind: Occasional Essays* (New York City: Penguin Books, 2010), p. 276 – emphasis in original. As a whole, the story is constructed as layers upon layers: we have an implicit narrator, who tells what the depressed protagonist has told her therapist, what she has told her friends on the phone and so on. In addition, we have the seemingly unending footnotes.
14. Franco "Bifo" Berardi, Félix Guattari. *Thought, Friendship, and Visionary Cartography* (London: Palgrave Macmillan, 2008), p. 130.
15. Thomas Fuchs, "Melancholia as a Desynchronization: Towards a Psychopathology of Interpersonal Time," in *Psychopathology* 34, 2001, p. 185.
16. Henri Lefebvre, *rhythanalysis. space time and everyday life*, trans. Stuart Elden (London: Continuum, 2004), p. 15.

17. Berardi, *Félix Guattari*, p. 128-129. See also the chapter on the refrain/ritornello in Gilles Deleuze and Félix Guattari, *A Thousand Plateaus*, trans. Brian Massumi (London: Continuum, 2004), pp. 342ff.

18. Jaspers, *General Psychopathology*, p. 64.

19. Ibid., p. 55.

20 Cf. René Rosfort and Giovanni Stanghellini, "Jaspers on Feelings and Affective States," in *Karl Jasper's Philosophy and Psychopathology*, ed. Thomas Fuchs et al. (New York: Springer, 2013), p. 166.

21. Wallace, *Brief Interviews with Hideous Men*, pp. 20-22; 22ff.; 86.

22. Ibid., p. 138.

23. Simon Baron-Cohen, "The Science of Evil," in *New York Times*, 6 June, 2011, http://www.nytimes.com/2011/06/07/science/14evil-excerpt.html?_r=0. See also: Franco "Bifo" Berardi, And: *Phenomenology of the End* (Los Angeles: Semiotext(e), 2015), pp. 16ff.).

24. For the most obvious example, see: Mary K. Holland, "The Art's Heart's Purpose": Braving the Narcissistic Loop of David Foster Wallace's *Infinite Jest*," in *Critique: Studies in Contemporary Fiction* 47, 2006. But the reference point for nearly all of these readings is, of course, Christopher Lasch, *The Culture of* Narcissism: *American Life in an Age of Diminishing Expectations* (New York: W.W. Norton & Company, 1979).

25. David Foster Wallace, *Infinite Jest* (New York: Black Ray Books, 2006), pp. 298; 521. For more on this particular topic, see: Stefan Hirt, *The Iron Bars of Freedom* (Stuttgart: *ibidem*-Verlag, 2008), p. 33.

26. David Foster Wallace, *This is Water* (Boston: Little, Brown and Company, 2009), p. 117. However, it is vital not to regard these "tiny skull-sized kingdoms," this pronounced narcissism, as a simple love of the self. The egoist subject

continuously undertakes a demarcation in relation to other subjects, whereas the narcissistic subject cannot clearly define his or her boundaries. According to German philosopher Byung-Chul Han this is precisely a symptom of a society in which all forms of negativity and alterity have disappeared. In a society of pure positivity, the Other (with a capital O) no longer exists, or if it does, merely as a reflection, a mirror image of the self. For Han, this means that today, love is in straitened circumstances, while, conversely, favorable conditions for depression abound (Byung-Chul Han, Müdigkeitsgesellschaft (Berlin: Verlag Matthes & Seitz Berlin, 2010), pp. 15ff.).

27. David Foster Wallace, *The Pale King* (New York: Black Ray Books, 2012), p. 96.

28. David Foster Wallace, *Everything and More* (New York: W.W. Norton & Company, 2010), p. 49.

29. Michael North is one of the readers of Wallace who has a very strong sense of the comedy of his works (Michael North, *Machine-Age Comedy* (Oxford: Oxford University Press, 2009), pp. 169ff.).

30. Ludwig Wittgenstein, *Philosophical Investigations*, trans. G. E. Anscombe et al. (Chichester: Wiley-Blackwell, 2009), p. 255; 57; 110.

31. David Foster Wallace, *Consider the Lobster. And Other Essays* (London: Abacus, 2007), p. 65.

32. Judith Butler, *Giving an Account of Oneself* (New York: Fordham Univ. Press, 2005), p. 32.

33. Wallace, *Infinite Jest*, p. 740.

34. Wallace, *Brief Interviews with Hideous Men,* p. 195.

35. Wallace, *Infinite Jest,* p. 73.

36. Ibid.

37. Ibid., p. 74.

38. David Foster Wallace, *The David Foster Wallace Reader* (New York: Back Bay Books, 2015), p. 10.

39. Ibid., p. 11.
40. Wallace, *Infinite Jest,* p. 74.
41. Ibid., p. 692.
42. Ibid., pp. 692-693.
43. James, *Varieties of Religious Experience*, p. 146.
44. Houellebecq, *Atomised,* pp. 99-100.
45. Wallace, *Infinite Jest,* p. 694.
46. Ibid., p. 694.
47. Ibid., p. 695.
48. Ibid., pp. 695-696.
49. Ibid., p. 72.
50. Ibid., p. 78 – emphasis in original.
51. Ibid., p. 75.
52. The title of both the film and the novel is, of course, taken from the scene in Shakespeare's *Hamlet,* where Hamlet exclaims: "Alas, poor Yorick! I knew him, Horatio: a fellow of infinite jest."
53. Ibid., p. 779.
54. Ibid., p. 696.
55. Ibid., pp. 76-78.
56. Ibid., pp. 222-223.
57. Cf. Fisher, *Capitalist Realism* 22.
58. Andrew Weil, *The Natural Mind: A new way of looking at drugs and the higher consciousness* (New York: Mariner Books, 1998), p. 9. What Weil and Wallace do not in any way share is Weil's romantic and rather dated conception of psychosis as something *positive*: "I am almost tempted," Weil writes at one point, "to call psychotics the evolutionary vanguard of our species." (Ibid., p. 182).
59. Lasch, *The Culture of Narcissism,* p. 99.
60. Ehrenberg, *The Weariness of the Self,* p. 12; 133.
61. Wallace, *Infinite Jest,* p. 203.
62. Wallace, *The Pale King,* p. 188 – my emphasis.
63. Lauren Berlant, *Cruel Optimism* (Durham: Duke University

Press, 2011), p. 24.

64. David Foster Wallace, *A Supposedly Fun Thing I'll Never Do Again* (Boston: Little, Brown and Company, 1997), p. 38.

65. North, *Machine-Age Comedy*, p. 174.

66. A great deal of mystery surrounds this film, which ostensibly exists in various versions (five or six). According to Joelle, she appears in two scenes in the lethally entertaining version (which is either *Infinite Jest V* or *Infinite Jest VI*). In addition to the scene with the revolving doors, there is a second in which Joelle, leaning into a crib where an infant lies, repeats the line "I am sorry, I am so so sorry" over and over again in a wobbly, blurred shot as if seen from the infant's point of view (Wallace, *Infinite Jest,* pp. 938-941). But her friend Molly suggests that the movie consists of another scene as well, in which a naked Joelle features as "some kind of maternal instantiation of the archetypal figure death," meanwhile explaining to the camera that "Death is always female, and that the female is always maternal. i.e. that the woman who kills you is always your next life's mother." (Ibid., p. 788).

67. Ibid., p. 347.

68. Félix Guattari, *Soft Subversions. Texts and Interviews 1977-1985,* Chet Wiener (Los Angeles: Semiotext(e), 2009), p. 158.

69. Natasha Dow Schull, *Addiction by design. Machine Gambling in Las Vegas* (Princeton: Princeton University Press, 2014), p. 2.

70. Ibid., p. 173.

71. Deleuze and Guattari, *A Thousand Plateaus*, p. 506.

72. Maurizio Lazzarato, *Signs and Machines. Capitalism and the Production of Subjectivity,* trans. Joshua David Jordan (Cambridge: The MIT Press, 2014), p. 27.

73. Félix Guattari, *The Anti-Œdipus Papers*, trans. Kélina Gotman (Cambridge: MIT Press, 2006), p. 79.

74. Wallace, *This is Water*, pp. 96-101.

75. Burn, *Conversations with David Foster Wallace*, p. 22.

76. Wallace, *Brief Interviews with Hideous Men*, pp. 293-4.

77. Ibid., 300-301.

78. Ibid., p. 301.

79. Ibid., p. 288.

80. Ibid., p. 318.

81. Ibid., p. 301.

82. Other critics have noted this dynamic. See for example: Boswell, *Understanding David Foster Wallace*, p. 196.

83. Søren Kierkegaard, *Works of Love (Kierkegaard's Writings, XVI)*, ed. and trans. Howard V. Hong and Edna Hong (Princeton: Princeton Univ. Press, 1998), p. 22.

84. Ibid.

85. Ibid., p. 222 – emphasis in original.

86. Ibid., p. 59.

87. Ibid., p. 58.

88. Ibid., p. 374.

89. Burn, *Conversations with David Foster Wallace*, p. 21.

90. Boswell, *Understanding David Foster Wallace*, p. 196.

91. Kierkegaard, *Works of Love*, p. 176.

92. Wallace, *Infinite Jest*, p. 860.

93. Kierkegaard, *Works of Love*, p. 186. Kierkegaard actually compares (pun intended) the act of comparing to an arrow flying through the air: As soon as it becomes aware of itself and of what it is doing, as soon as it "dwells" on itself and begins comparing one state with another, it falls to the ground (ibid., p. 182). One might think of the prototypical scene in a cartoon in which a character runs at full speed beyond the edge of a cliff and according to the law of gravity ought to fall, but does not, remaining suspended in mid-air. However, the moment the character looks down, comparing its own situation to the requirements of physical laws, *then* it immediately crashes to the ground.

94. Ibid., p. 185.

95. N. Katherine Hayles, "The Illusion of Autonomy and the Fact of Recursivity: Virtual Ecologies, Entertainment and *Infinite Jest*," in *New Literary History* 30, 1999, p. 693.

96. Wallace, *Infinite Jest*, p. 345.

97. Levinas, *Time and the Other*, p. 75.

98. Jaspers, *General Psychopathology*, p. 792; 805.

99. Ibid., p. 792.

100. Wallace Stevens, *Opus Posthumous* (New York: Random House, 1982), p. 163. Coincidentally, these particular lines by Stevens are not only cited by Simon Critchley (Simon Critchley, *The Faith of the Faithless. Experiments in Political Theology* (London/New York: Verso, 2014), p. 91), but also by Boswell (Boswell, *Understanding David Foster Wallace*, p. 147).

101. Wallace, *Infinite Jest*, p. 773 – my emphasis.

102. Nussbaum, *Poetic Justice*, pp. 66-68.

103. Wallace, *Infinite Jest*, p. 379.

104. Ibid., p. 696.

105. Kierkegaard, *Works of Love*, p. 42.

106. Wallace, *Infinite Jest*, p. 107.

107. Wallace, *This is Water*, p. 121.

108. Susan Sontag, *Styles of Radical Will* (New York: Picador, 2002), p. 3.

109. James, *Varieties of Religious Experience*, p. 113.

110. Ibid., p. 162.

Chapter 3. Shooting the ambulance? – Claire Fontaine

1. The use of pronouns poses something of a problem, but I shall alternate between the plural of the two artists that make up the duo (them), and the singular of the artist as an interface (her).

2. Claire Fontaine, *Human Strike Has Already Begun & Other Writings* (Berlin: Mute Books, 2013), pp. 38-39.

3. Maybe this is why very little has been written about Claire Fontaine, at least within academic and scholarly circles – with Hal Foster as one exception (see his essay "None Reasons Why the Avant-Garde Shouldn't Give up" in the catalog *Foreigners Everywhere* (Köln: Walther König, 2013), pp. 144-159). However, several useful interviews do exist. In one of them, a dialog between Claire Fontaine and Bernard Blistène and Nicolas Liucci-Goutnikov, the latter remarks "[i]f, as I believe, the artwork only has accounts to settle with the history of its own genre, the dissensus it engenders must have to do with what it is," and that the work "seems to oscillate between utopia and melancholy" (*Foreigners Everywhere*, p. 40; 48). In any case, it is fair to say that Claire Fontaine is an artist who has a strained relationship to herself as an artist, as well as to the very institution(s) of art, even if she has never left it.

4. Andrew Ross, *Creditocracy: And The Case For Debt Refusal* (New York: OR Books, 2014).

5. David Graeber, *Debt – the first 5000 years*, (Brooklyn: Melville House, 2011), p. 70.

6. Wolfgang Streeck, *Buying Time – The Delayed Crisis of Democratic Capitalism* (London: Verso, 2014), p. 165. For more on Streeck's take on debt in the Southern part of the Eurozone, see: pp. 343ff.

7. Christian Marazzi, *The Violence of Financial Capitalism*, trans. Kristina Lebedeva (Los Angeles: Semiotext(e), 2010), p. 10.

8. Kojin Karatani, *Transcritique: On Kant and Marx*, Trans. Sabu Kohso (Cambridge, MA: MIT Press, 2005), p. 220.

9. International Monetary Fund, "Fiscal Monitor: Debt. Use It Wisely," 2016, http://www.imf.org/external/pubs/ft/fm/2016/02/pdf/fm1602.pdf. The IMF-blogpost can be found here: https://blogs.imf.org/2016/10/05/big-bad-actors-a-glo bal-view-of-debt/.

10. Post-crisis development in Southern Europe needs little narration here. The back and forth between Greece and the IMF and EU is, for example, a story in itself: the bailout loans, the austerity measures imposed on Greece in return, Alexis Tsipras and Yanis Varoufakis demanding debt relief, Angela Merkel and the European Banks refusing etc.

11. https://biennale4.thessalonikibiennale.gr/content/claire-fontaine.

12. Andrew Culp and Ricky Crano, "Claire Fontaine. Giving shape to painful things," in *Radical Philosophy* 175, 2012, p. 46.

13. Ibid.

14. I caution the reader not to be too parochial about my use of the word avant-garde in this context. I am going to pretend that I will be able to unravel all the complexities hidden in the history of the avant-garde, nor do I wish to engage in lengthy discussion of the canonical texts on this subject (for instance, Peter Bürger's influential book *Theory of the Avant-Garde* from 1974). I am simply going to operate under the assumption that the project of the avant-garde was characterized by the attempt to unite art and life and by a general belief in the future, or, rather, a belief in the capacity of avant-garde art to initiate and create a new and better future.

15. Anthony Huberman, "Claire Fontaine," *BOMB Magazine* 105, 2008, http://bombmagazine.org/article/3177/claire-fontaine.

16. Jerry Saltz, "Musings on the Mutinies to Come," in *Village Voice*, 11 October 2005, http://www.villagevoice.com/arts/musings-on-the-mutinies-to-come-7137097.

17. Maurizio Lazzarato, *The Making of the Indebted Man. An Essay on the Neoliberal Condition*, trans. Joshua David Jordan (Los Angeles: Semiotext(e), 2011), p. 52.

18. Friedrich Nietzsche, *On the Genealogy of Morality*, trans.

Carol Diethe (Cambridge: Cambridge University Press, 1997), p. 39.

19. Ibid., p. 36.
20. Lazzarato, *The Making of the Indebted Man*, p. 55.
21. Ibid., p. 88 – my emphasis.
22. John Gathergood, "Debt and Depression: Causal Links and Social Norm Effects," in *The Economic Journal* 122:56, 2012.
23. H. Meltzer et al., "Personal debt and suicidal ideation," in *Psychological Medicine* 41, 2011 – quoted from abstract.
24. David Stuckler and Sanjay Basu, *The Body Economic. Why Austerity Kills. Recessions, Budget Battles, and the Politics of Life and Death* (New York: Basic Books, 2013), p. 127.
25. Ibid., p. xviii.
26. It should be noted in passing that the incident is not only reminiscent of Dimitris Christoulas but also of the German pilot Andreas Lubitz, who in March 2015 deliberately crashed an aircraft in the French Alps, killing all 144 passengers and the six crew members on board. One might even include in this tragic tradition Seung-Hui Cho, the depressed American teenager – born in South Korea – who in 2007 shot and killed 32 people before committing suicide at Virginia Polytechnic Institute and State University in what was to become known as the Virginia Tech Massacre. Like many before him, Cho had a history of mental health problems, including a diagnosis of a major depressive disorder. In one of his new books *Heroes. Mass murder and suicide,* Franco "Bifo" Berardi writes about such persons as Joseph Stack, Andreas Lubitz and Seung-Hui Cho – although only the latter is treated specifically in the book – calling them, quite provocatively, heroes. This claim is to be taken in a very specific sense, however: "I write about spectacular murderous suicides," Berardi writes at the outset, "because these killers are the extreme manifestation of one of the main trends of our age. I see them as heroes

of an age of nihilism and spectacular stupidity: the age of financial capitalism." (Franco "Bifo" Berardi, *Heroes. Mass murder and suicide* (London: Verso, 2015), p. 3). Berardi's concern here is the point at which the psychopathologies of contemporary capitalism are turned outwards; the point at which depression becomes aggressive and violent; the point at which suicide is transformed into mass murder.

27. They have stated in an interview that "the suicide letter is interesting because Stack's confusion makes his final gesture understandable." (Ossian Ward, "Just who on earth is Claire Fontaine?" in *TimeOut London*, 3 February 2011, http://www.timeout.com/london/art/just-who-on-earth-is-claire-fontaine).

28. As part of my research for this chapter, I took a trip to Frankfurt in 2014 (and wrote about it in the Danish newspaper *Information*). The present scene takes this trip as its point of departure. No coincidence, perhaps, that I came across a so-called *Spielothek* and the European Central Bank on my route from the airport to the art museum. A culture of instant gratification and the politics of necessity, or infinite jest and infinite debt; this is the dual reality that the works in the exhibition confronted in various ways.

29. The two other works are *Untitled* from 2008 – an amputated arm made of latex, holding its fist closed and carrying a Rolex Submariner watch with a Pepsi-Cola dial – and *Untitled* (Tennis Ball Sculpture) from 2010 – consisting of hundreds of tennis balls lying around on the floor of the gallery floor. The balls have been sliced open and filled with various objects – pencils, toothbrushes, cell phone chargers. Reportedly, things are smuggled into American prisons in this way...

30. Karl Marx: *Capital. Volume 1, Marx & Engels: Collected Works, Volume 35*, trans. Samuel Moore and Edward Aveling (Chadwell Heath: Lawrence & Wishart, 2010), p. 140; 163.

31. Moishe Postone, *Time, labor, and social domination. A reinterpretation of Marx's critical theory* (Cambridge: Cambridge University Press, 1993), pp. 181-182.

32. Bernard Stiegler, *For a New Critique of Political Economy*, trans. Daniel Ross (Cambridge: Polity Press, 2010), p. 68.

33. Joseph Vogl, "Capital and Money are Profane Gods," in *The European*, 20 November 2011, http://www.theeuropean-magazine.com/371-vogl-joseph/370-the-spectre-of-capital.

34. Latour, "On some of the affects of capitalism."

35. I quote here from a gallery text for Claire Fontaine's first solo exhibition in Rome at Galeria T293 in Spring 2012 (www.t293.it/exhibitions/claire-fontaine/).

36. Visitors to galleries exhibiting Claire Fontaine's works are often met by such one-liners before they have even entered the gallery space. Often the neon signs are placed at the very entrance, ensuring that the visitors really cannot miss them. Most of the signs are blue, red and/or white, some flash, others do not. In most cases it is clear *what* the utterances are referring to; what is less clear is *who* the senders and perceived receivers of the utterances are. To put it in dusted structuralist terms: There is an abyss between the *énoncé* and the *énonciation,* between what is said and the act or process of saying it. There is also, more often than not, no decipherable subject behind the enunciations. Again, this has to do with the fact that some, if not all, of the neon signs are ready-mades: *Past Present Future* presumably reproduces a sign from a clairvoyant shop in New York. As for the sign *Please God Make Tomorrow Better*, it is an open question, who the subject behind this sentence is? Is it the voice of financial capital – Lehman Brothers perhaps – or the voice of a depressed person, or a revolutionary prayer stemming from Claire Fontaine herself?

37. www.biennale4.thessalonikibiennale.gr/content/claire-fontaine.

38. Lazzarato, *The Making of the Indebted Man*, p. 46.
39. Claire Fontaine, *Untitled (Why your psychology sucks)*, video, 2015.
40. Ibid. – emphasis mine.
41. Mark Fisher, "Good for nothing," in *The Occupied Times*, 19 March 2014, https://theoccupiedtimes.org/?p=12841.
42. In a very apt phrase, Carl Cederström and André Spicer call this "an insourcing of responsibility" (Carl Cederström and André Spicer, *The Wellness Syndrome* (Cambridge: Polity Press, 2015), p. 13).
43. The Invisible Committee, *To Our Friends*, trans. Robert Hurley (Los Angeles: Semiotext(e), 2015), p. 163.
44. The Invisible Committee, *The Coming Insurrection* (Los Angeles: Semiotext(e), 2008), pp. 49-51.
45. Ben Davis, *9.5 Theses on Art and Class* (Chicago: Haymarket Books, 2013), p. 25.
46. Realism Working Group: "Historical fiction as realism" (interview with Claire Fontaine), year unkown and unpaginated, https://realismworkinggroup.org/interview-with-claire-fontaine/.
47. Bernadette Corporation, *Get Rid of Yourself*, video, 2003. The film is available here: www.vimeo.com/25952876.
48. The Invisible Committee, *The Coming Insurrection*, p. 34.
49. Claire Fontaine, *Human Strike Has Already Begun & Other Writings*, p. 29.
50. Walter B. Rideout, *The Radical Novel in the United States, 1900-1954* (New York: Columbia University Press, 1992), p. 172.
51. Boltanski and Chiapello write that the total strike days in France annually averaged 4,000,000 in the years 1971-1975 and less than half a million in 1992 (Boltanski and Chiapello, *The New Spirit of Capitalism*, p. 169).
52. Claire Fontaine, *Human Strike Has Already Begun & Other Writings*, p. 39.

53. Ibid., p. 55.
54. Fulvia Carnevale and John Kelsey, "Grève Humaine (Interrompue). Fulvia Carnevale and John Kelsey in conversation," http://secularmiracle.com/the_workers_installing/the_work/FCarnevale-JKelsey-ENG.pdf.
55. Claire Fontaine, *Human Strike Has Already Begun & Other Writings*, p. 29.
56. Davis, *9.5 Theses on Art and Class*, p. 14.
57. Ibid., p. 19.
58. Claire Fontaine, "Ready-Made Artists and Human Strike: A few Clarifications," 2005, http://frontdeskapparatus.com/wp/wp-content/uploads/2012/10/Fontaine_Readymade.pdf.
59. Boris Groys, "On Art Activism," (unpaginated), *e-flux* 56, June 2014, http://www.e-flux.com/journal/56/60343/on-art-activism/.
60. Hito Steyerl, *The Wretched of the Screen* (Berlin: Sternberg Press, 2012), p. 110.
61. Patricia Reed, "Seven Prescriptions," in *#Accelerate: The Accelerationist Reader*, ed. Robin Mackay and Armen Avanessian (Falmouth: Urbanomic, 2014), p. 524. Considering the global world as a whole and the spread of precarious working conditions, this is obviously a qualified truth that only applies to some very specific contexts in the Western world; or at least, this is the myth sold to a section of the de-industrialized working class.
62. Groys, "On Art Activism."
63. Ibid.
64. Carnevale and Kelsey, "Grève Humaine (Interrompue)."
65. Claire Fontaine, "Ready-Made Artists and Human Strike: A few Clarifications."
66. Now is as good a time as any to refer the reader to other investigations into the relation between what Fredric Jameson in his famous article from 1997 called "Culture

and Finance Capital," in particular the relation between culture and debt. See: Mark W. Rectanus, "Artists, debt, and global activism," in *Finance and Society*, 2:1, 2016; Leigh Claire La Berge and Dehlia Hannah, "Debt Aesthetics: Medium Specificity and Social Practice in the Work of Cassie Thornton," in *Postmodern Culture* 25:2, 2015; Yates McKee, "~~DEBT~~: Occupy, Postcontemporary Art, and the Aesthetics of Debt Resistance," in *South Atlantic Quarterly*, 112:4, 2013; Annie McClanahan, *Dead Pledges: Debt, Crisis, and Twenty-First Century Culture* (Stanford: Stanford University Press, 2016).

67. Lazzarato, *The Making of the Indebted Man*, pp. 46-47.
68. As Walker Percy writes in his mock self-help book *Lost in the Cosmos*: "You are depressed because you have every reason to be depressed. No member of the other two million species which inhabit the earth—and who are luckily exempt from depression—would fail to be depressed if it lived the life you lead. You live in a deranged age—more deranged than usual, because despite great scientific and technological advances, man has not the faintest idea of who he is or what he is doing. Begin with the reverse hypothesis, like Copernicus and Einstein. You are depressed because you should be. You are entitled to your depression. In fact, you'd be deranged if you were not depressed. Consider the only adults who are never depressed: chuckleheads, California surfers, and fundamentalist Christians who believe they have had a personal encounter with Jesus and are saved for once and all. Would you trade your depression to become any of these?" (Walker Percy, *Lost in the Cosmos. The Last Self-Help Book* (New York: Picador, 2000), p. 76).
69. Cf. Jan Verwoert, *Tell Me What You Want, What You Really, Really Want* (Berlin: Sternberg Press, 2011), pp. 13ff.

Chapter 4. Happiness and the end of the world as we know it – Lars von Trier's *Melancholia*

1. As far as clinical terms go, I shall speak about Justine's depression, even though the movie is called *Melancholia*. The reason for using the concept of depression instead of that of melancholia should be clear from the introduction to this book and will be taken for granted in what follows. A couple of times, however, given the title of the movie and the vocabulary it generally employs, I have found myself compelled to use the word melancholia to refer to Justine's condition, but the conceptual meaning remains the same.

2. It is, of course, also impossible to ignore the allusion to the pre-Raphaelite painting of Ophelia by John Everett Millais (1851/1852).

3. Henri Bergson, Laughter. *An Essay on the Meaning of the Comic*, trans. Cloudesley Shovell Henry Brereton (Rockville: Arc Manor, 2008), p. 36.

4. Sianne Ngai and Lauren Berlant, "Comedy Has Issues," in *Critical Inquiry* 43, 2017, p. 234.

5. Fuchs, "Melancholia as a Desynchronization," p. 179.

6. Martin Heidegger, *Being and Time*, trans. John Macquarrie and Edward Robinson (Oxford: Blackwell, 1962), pp. 370ff.

7. Byung-Chul Han, *Agonie des Eros* (Berlin: Verlag Matthes & Seitz Berlin, 2012), p. 23 – emphasis in original.

8. William Davies, *The Happiness Industry: How the Government and Big Business Sold Us Well-Being* (London/New York: Verso, 2015), p. 3.

9. Cf. www.theguardian.com/politics/2010/nov/14/david-ca meron-wellbeing-inquiry. For more on this issue, see: Carl Cederström and André Spicer, *The Wellness Syndrome*, pp. 75ff.

10. Davies, *The Happiness Industry,* p. 5 (see also pp. 20; 41-69).

11. World Economic Forum, *The Wellness Imperative – Creating More Effective Organizations.* Cologny/Geneva, 2010,

http://www3.weforum.org/docs/WEF_HE_Wellness ImperativeCreatingMoreEffectiveOrganizations_Report _2010.pdf.

12. Alenka Zupančič, The Odd One In: On Comedy (Cambridge, MA: MIT Press, 2008), p. 5.

13. Barbara Ehrenreich, Smile or Die. How Positive Thinking Fooled America and the World (London: Granta Books, 2009), p. 8.

14. Cederström and Spicer, The Wellness Syndrome, p. 29; 13.

15. Giorgio Agamben, Means without End, trans. Cesare Casarino and Vincenzo Binetti (Minneapolis: University of Minnesota Press, 2000), p. 4.

16. Heidegger, Being and Time, pp. 304ff.

17. Berardi, The Soul at Work, p. 92.

18. Friedrich Nietzsche, Thus Spoke Zarathustra, trans. Adrian Del Caro (Cambridge: Cambridge University Press, 2006), p. 10.

19. Francis Fukuyama, "The End of History?" in The National Interest 16, 1989, p. 18.

20. Steven Shaviro, "Melancholia or, The Romantic Anti-Sublime," in Sequence 1.1, 2012, pp. 6-7, http://reframe. sussex.ac.uk/sequence/files/2012/12/MELANCHOLIA-or-The-Romantic-Anti-Sublime-SEQUENCE-1.1-2012-Steven-Shaviro.pdf; Mark B. Sandberg, "Apocalypse Then and Now: Verdens Undergang (1916) and Melancholia (2011)," in European Journal of Scandinavian Studies 46(1), 2016, p. 9.

21. Fisher, Capitalist Realism, p. 2.

22. Berardi, After the Future, p. 126; Fredric Jameson, The Cultural Turn. Selected Writings on the Postmodern, 1983-1998 (London/New York: Verso, 1998), p. 91.

23. I am deliberately avoiding the concept of the Anthropocene, since the term is heavily disputed. As Andreas Malm has stated, "[b]laming all of humanity for climate change lets capitalism off the hook" (Andreas Malm, "The Anthropocene

Myth," in *Jacobin Magazine,* 2015, https://www.jacobinmag. com/2015/03/anthropocene-capitalism-climate-change/). See also, T. J. Demos' *Against the Anthropocene,* the title of which says it all; Jason W. Moore's *Capitalism in the Web of Life. Ecology and the Accumulation of Capital,* a book that develops and subscribes to a notion of the *capitalocene;* and Donna Haraway's *Staying with the Trouble,* which proposes the term the *Chthulucene* as a conceptual alternative to the Anthropocene.

24. Sylvere Lotringer, "The Last Political Scene – Sylvere Lotringer in conversation with Heather Davis and Etienne Turpin," in *Art in the Anthropocene,* ed. Heather Davis and Etienne Turpin (London: Open Humanities Press, 2015), p. 374.

25. Claire Colebrook, "Anthropocene," in *Speculations ("The future is _____"),* ed. Sarah Resnick. (New York: Triple Canopy, 2015), 143.

26. Claire Colebrook, "Extinction," in *Speculations ("The future is _____"),* ed. Sarah Resnick. (New York: Triple Canopy, 2015), 45.

27. Shaviro, "Melancholia or, The Romantic Anti-Sublime," p. 13.

28. Sandberg, "Apocalypse Then and Now," pp. 109-110.

29. "Von Trier's own uneasiness with Melancholia may well stem from the fact that — for perhaps the only time in his entire career — he has made a film that is non-ironic, heartfelt, and sincere." (Shaviro, "Melancholia or, The Romantic Anti-Sublime," p. 9).

30. Quoted in: Sandberg, "Apocalypse Then and Now," p. 116.

31. Shaviro, "Melancholia or, The Romantic Anti-Sublime," p. 13.

32. Quentin Meillassoux, *After Finitude. An Essay on the Contingency of Necessity,* trans. Ray Brassier (New York/ London: Bloomsbury Academic, 2010), p. 116.

33. Shaviro, "Melancholia or, The Romantic Anti-Sublime," p. 10.
34. Ibid.
35. Ibid., 11.
36. Sandberg, "Apocalypse Then and Now," p. 116.
37. Arthur Schopenhauer, *The World as Will and Representation*, trans. E. F. J. Payne (New York: Dover, 1969), p. 412. Eugene Thacker also quotes this passage (Eugene Thacker, *In the Dust of Our Planet. Horror of Philosophy vol. 1* (London: Zero Books, 2011), p. 19.)
38. Ernst Bloch, *The Principle of Hope*, trans. Neville Plaice et al. (Cambridge, MA: MIT Press, 1995), p. 1376).
39. Eve Kosofsky Sedgwick, *Touching Feeling. Affect, Pedagogy, Performativity* (Durham: Duke University Press), p. 133.
40. Ibid., 13.
41. Fisher, *Ghosts of My Life*, p. 61.
42. Sedgwick, *Touching Feeling*, p. 147.
43. Sandberg, "Apocalypse Then and Now," p. 13.
44. Shaviro, "Melancholia or, The Romantic Anti-Sublime," p. 10.
45. Freud, "Mourning and Melancholia," p. 206. Justine's own statement is not the only thing that leads scholars and critics in this direction. Lars von Trier himself entertained the idea in an interview, in which he quite coquettishly mentions how his analyst told him "that melancholics will be more level-headed than ordinary people in a disastrous situation, partly because they can say: 'What did I tell you?'." (Nils Thorsen, "Longing for the End of It All," interview with Lars von Trier in Melancholia Press Kit, 2011, http://www.melancholiathemovie.com/#_interview).
46. According to Jean-Pierre Dupuy this is precisely how we – meaning humanity as such – should approach any future catastrophe: As something that has *already happened*. As something that could not *not* have taken place. In works such as *Pour un catastrophisme éclairé: Quand l'impossible*

est certain (2004) and *Petite métaphysique des tsunamis* (2005), Dupuy thus advances the argument that a coming catastrophe should be perceived in the future anterior, as something that will have been.

47. In the words of Slavoj Žižek, the cynic is "the victim of the most radical self-deception...the cynic misses the actuality of the appearance itself." (Slavoj Žižek, *Event* (New York: Melville House, 2014), p. 89). What the cynic fails to see is that illusions and symbolic fictions are not necessarily, nor only, strategies for *escaping* reality, but can be strategies for *transforming* this very reality.

48. Stevens, *Opus Posthumous*, p. 163.

49. In an article on von Trier's *Melancholia*, Sylvia Chong dubs the building of the magic cave as Justine's "concession" to Leo, and states that the tipi "barely" constitutes even "the pretense of a shelter." (Sylvia Chong, "The illusion of a future: hopelessness in contemporary cinema," in *Hopelessness: Developmental, Cultural, and Clinical Realms,* ed. Salman Akhtar and Mary Kay O'Neil (London: Routledge, 2014), p. 115). However, this is precisely my point: The tipi is not to be so readily dismissed, particularly not because it is *not* a shelter. The "pretense" and the make-believe of the magic cave is what makes the final scene a hopeful one; the illusion of a future does not reinforce hopelessness; rather, it is what hope is made of.

50. Jonathan Lear, *Radical Hope. Ethics in the Face of Cultural Devastation* (Cambridge: Harvard University Press, 2006), p. 103.

51. Bonnie Honig, "Public Things: Jonathan Lear's *Radical Hope*, Lars von Trier's *Melancholia*, and the Democratic Need," in *Political Research Quarterly* Vol. 68(3), 2015, p. 630.

52. James Martel, "Against Thinning and Teleology: Politics and Objects in the Face of Catastrophe in Lear and von

Trier," in *Political Research Quarterly* Vol. 68(3), 2015, p. 644.

53. Kierkegaard, *Sickness unto Death,* p. 38.

54. Bloch, *The Principle of Hope,* p. 3.

55. Ibid., p. 445.

56. In a recent article, Rebecca Coleman has developed the useful concept of a hopeful pessimism, which is not too dissimilar to the one deployed here: "In Berlant's terms, hopeful pessimism can be understood as a mood that involves being worn out by debt and austerity and a resistance to this wearing out." (Rebecca Coleman, "Austerity Futures: Debt, Temporality and (Hopeful) Pessimism as an Austerity Mood," in *New Formations* 87, 2016, p. 100).

57. Bloch, *The Principle of Hope,* p. 446.

58. It was originally to be called Träume *vom* besseren Leben (Dreams of a Better Life).

59. Bloch, *The Principle of Hope,* p. 223.

60. Jürgen Moltmann, *Theology of Hope,* trans. James W. Leitch (Minneapolis: Fortress Press, 1993), p. 25.

61. Bloch, *The Principle of Hope,* p. 315.

62. Ibid., p. 17.

Epilogue (three songs and three paradoxes)

1. Kierkegaard, *Either/Or Vol 1,* pp. 20-21.

2. Søren Kierkegaard, *Concluding Unscientific Postscript to Philosophical Fragments. Vol. I,* ed. and trans. Howard V. Hong and Edna H. Hong (Princeton: Princeton University Press, 1992)., pp. 513-514.

3. Lauren Berlant, "Austerity, Precarity, Awkwardness," 2011, http://supervalentthought. files.wordpress.com/2011/12/ berlant-aaa-2011final.pdf.

4. Moltmann, *Theology of Hope,* p. 23.

5. Bloch, *The Principle of Hope,* p. 445.

CULTURE, SOCIETY & POLITICS

Contemporary culture has eliminated the concept and public figure of the intellectual. A cretinous anti-intellectualism presides, cheer-led by hacks in the pay of multinational corporations who reassure their bored readers that there is no need to rouse themselves from their stupor. Zer0 Books knows that another kind of discourse – intellectual without being academic, popular without being populist – is not only possible: it is already flourishing. Zer0 is convinced that in the unthinking, blandly consensual culture in which we live, critical and engaged theoretical reflection is more important than ever before.

If you have enjoyed this book, why not tell other readers by posting a review on your preferred book site.

Recent bestsellers from Zero Books are:

In the Dust of This Planet
Horror of Philosophy vol. 1
Eugene Thacker
In the first of a series of three books on the Horror of Philosophy, *In the Dust of This Planet* offers the genre of horror as a way of thinking about the unthinkable.
Paperback: 978-1-84694-676-9 ebook: 978-1-78099-010-1

Capitalist Realism
Is there no alternative?
Mark Fisher
An analysis of the ways in which capitalism has presented itself as the only realistic political-economic system.
Paperback: 978-1-84694-317-1 ebook: 978-1-78099-734-6

Rebel Rebel
Chris O'Leary
David Bowie: every single song. Everything you want to know, everything you didn't know.
Paperback: 978-1-78099-244-0 ebook: 978-1-78099-713-1

Cartographies of the Absolute
Alberto Toscano, Jeff Kinkle
An aesthetics of the economy for the twenty-first century.
Paperback: 978-1-78099-275-4 ebook: 978-1-78279-973-3

Malign Velocities
Accelerationism and Capitalism
Benjamin Noys
Long listed for the Bread and Roses Prize 2015, *Malign Velocities* argues against the need for speed, tracking acceleration as the symptom of the ongoing crises of capitalism.
Paperback: 978-1-78279-300-7 ebook: 978-1-78279-299-4

Meat Market
Female Flesh under Capitalism
Laurie Penny
A feminist dissection of women's bodies as the fleshy fulcrum of capitalist cannibalism, whereby women are both consumers and consumed.
Paperback: 978-1-84694-521-2 ebook: 978-1-84694-782-7

Poor but Sexy
Culture Clashes in Europe East and West
Agata Pyzik
How the East stayed East and the West stayed West.
Paperback: 978-1-78099-394-2 ebook: 978-1-78099-395-9

Romeo and Juliet in Palestine
Teaching Under Occupation
Tom Sperlinger
Life in the West Bank, the nature of pedagogy and the role of a
university under occupation.
Paperback: 978-1-78279-637-4 ebook: 978-1-78279-636-7

Sweetening the Pill
or How We Got Hooked on Hormonal Birth Control
Holly Grigg-Spall
Has contraception liberated or oppressed women? *Sweetening
the Pill* breaks the silence on the dark side of hormonal
contraception.
Paperback: 978-1-78099-607-3 ebook: 978-1-78099-608-0

Why Are We The Good Guys?
Reclaiming your Mind from the Delusions of Propaganda
David Cromwell
A provocative challenge to the standard ideology that Western
power is a benevolent force in the world.
Paperback: 978-1-78099-365-2 ebook: 978-1-78099-366-9

Readers of ebooks can buy or view any of these bestsellers by
clicking on the live link in the title. Most titles are published
in paperback and as an ebook. Paperbacks are available in
traditional bookshops. Both print and ebook formats are available
online.
Find more titles and sign up to our readers' newsletter
at http://www.johnhuntpublishing.com/culture-and-politics
Follow us on Facebook
at https://www.facebook.com/ZeroBooks
and Twitter at https://twitter.com/Zer0Books